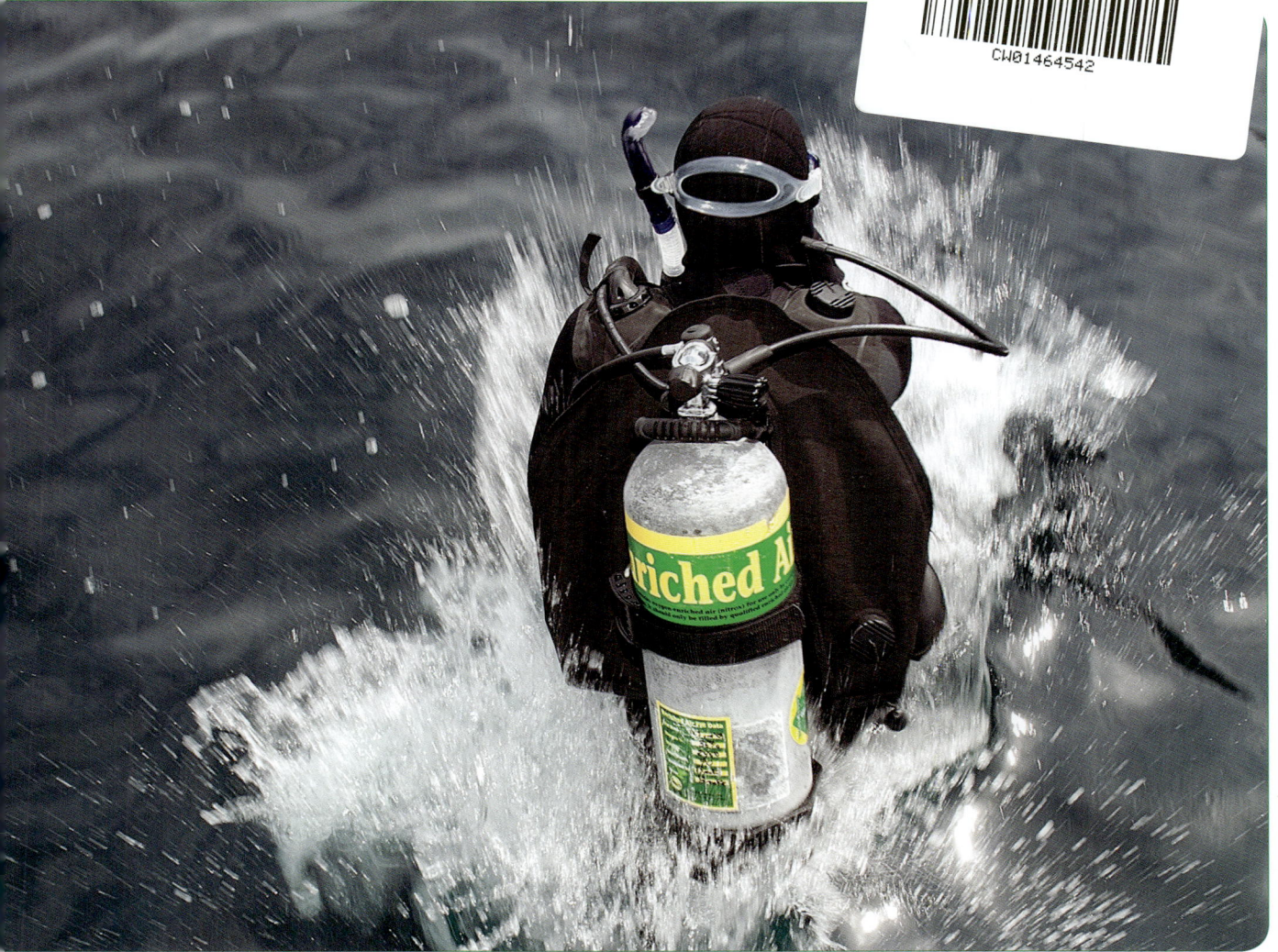

ENRICHED
AIR DIVER
MANUAL

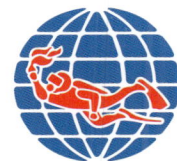

PADI
padi.com

Acknowledgments

PADI Would Like to Acknowledge

Professor Des Gorman, BSc, MBchB (Auckland), FAFOM, PhD, Head, Occupational Medicine, School of Medicine, University of Auckland, Auckland, New Zealand; Former President, South Pacific Underwater Medicine Society; Director, Occupational Diving and Hyperbaric Medicine, Royal New Zealand Navy;

and **Chris J. Acott**, MBBS, DipDHM, FFARACS, Diving & Hyperbaric Medicine Unit, Royal Adelaide Hospital, Adelaide, South Australia for their scientific and medical expertise in the development of PADI's enriched air nitrox programs.

A Special Dedication to Kenneth Donald, DSC, OBE, QP, DSc, MA, MD, FRCP, FRCPE, FRSE, Professor Emeritus of Medicine, Edinburgh University, acknowledging his groundbreaking research, 1942-1945, on the effects of oxygen on divers, which has benefited us all.

Development, Writing, Consultation and Review

Mark Caney, Pascal Dietrich, Al Hornsby, Brigit Jager, John Kinsella, Jean-Claude Monachon, Steve Mortell, Suzanne Pleydell, Drew Richardson EdD, Julie Taylor Sanders, Karl Shreeves, Bob Wohlers

Design and Production

Kristen Core

PADI® Enriched Air Diver *Manual*

Published by PADI
30151 Tomas
Rancho Santa Margarita, CA 92688-2125

ISBN 978-1-878663-85-6

Printed in USA

Product No. 70460 (Rev. 12/11) Version 1.01

Table of Contents

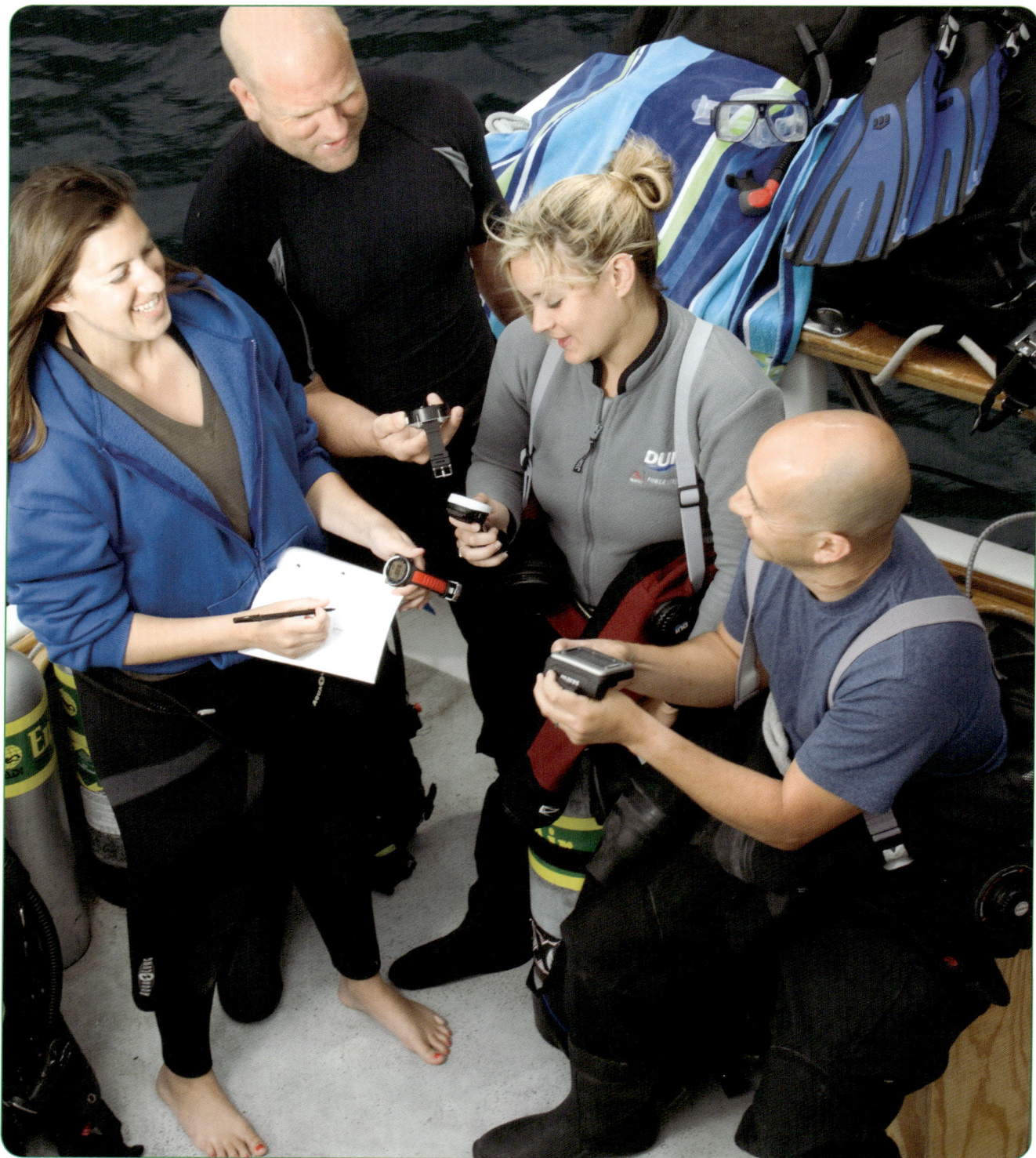

Introduction

Since its introduction into mainstream recreational diving in the mid 1990s, enriched air nitrox (EANx) has become established as a tool for increasing no stop (no decompression) dive time. While you once had to search to find a dive computer that you can set to use with EANx, today, virtually all dive computers available are capable of calculating nitrox dives. Combining enriched air nitrox with dive computers simplifies EANx dive planning and control. It maximizes your no stop dive time, yet helps you remain well within the limits.

At its introduction, enriched air nitrox diving required you to use special tables so you could determine your no stop dive time – no decompression limit. Some of these provided equivalent depths to use on tables developed for air, and others were tables written for EANx – with each blend requiring a different table. You used yet other tables to calculate your oxygen exposure (which isn't really an issue in recreational diving using air). Today, using tables is the exception rather than the rule. The rise of the EANx compatible dive computers has made the need for using tables with nitrox almost obsolete.

The PADI Enriched Air Diver course addresses the way recreational divers dive nitrox in the 21st century – with dive computers. In this course, you'll learn the benefits, potential problems, equipment considerations and other information you need to dive enriched air nitrox with an EANx dive computer. You'll also learn some simple, but important, skills to understand.

By successfully completing this course, you'll qualify for the PADI Enriched Air Diver certification. This certification means that you're qualified to buy and rent EANx dive gear, and to make and plan enriched air nitrox dives using an EANx compatible dive computer.

Special Activities and Enriched Air Diver

One reason that enriched air is so popular is that it's useful for almost all your dives. Regardless of what you love to do underwater, EANx gives you more dive time – more time to do what you love doing. There are a few activities, however, that *particularly* benefit from being a PADI Enriched Air Diver.

PADI Deep Diver – Deep diving (below 18 metres/60 feet) is adventurous, but the deeper you go, the shorter your no stop time. Although enriched air has some depth restrictions (more about this later), it has longer no decompression limits than air does. This helps offset the short no stop times you have on a deeper dive, so that you can stay down longer and still remain well within the limits.

PADI Digital Underwater Photographer – In the days of film, you had at most 36 pictures before you had to surface to reload. With digital imaging, this limit's gone. Having more dive time lets you take maximum advantage of your digital camera's capabilities.

PADI Dry Suit Diver – In moderately cool climates, diving dry means diving longer because you stay comfortable. Especially on repetitive dives, your no stop dive time limits your dives instead of how long you stay comfortable. Using EANx lets you benefit from the superior insulation you get from your dry suit. So, if you have a dry suit, you also want to have an enriched air dive computer and the PADI Enriched Air Diver certification.

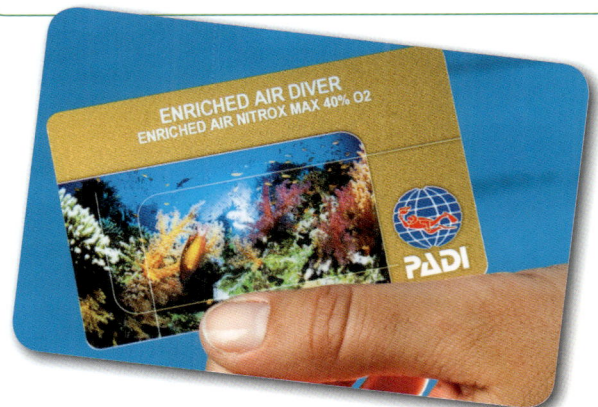

By successfully completing this course, you'll qualify for the PADI Enriched Air Diver certification.

Watch for These Symbols

⚠️ Pay particular attention when you see this symbol because the noted information has a strong bearing on your safety.

🔷 This symbol tells you where you can look for more information on various topics.

Learn more...

Important

⚠️ Although you can learn the basic principles for diving with enriched air nitrox using an EANx compatible computer by reading this manual, nothing replaces training and certification by a certified PADI Enriched Air Instructor. Reputable enriched air fill stations will not rent enriched air cylinders or fill enriched air cylinders unless you can show them an enriched air certification.

Continue Your ADVENTURE Today!

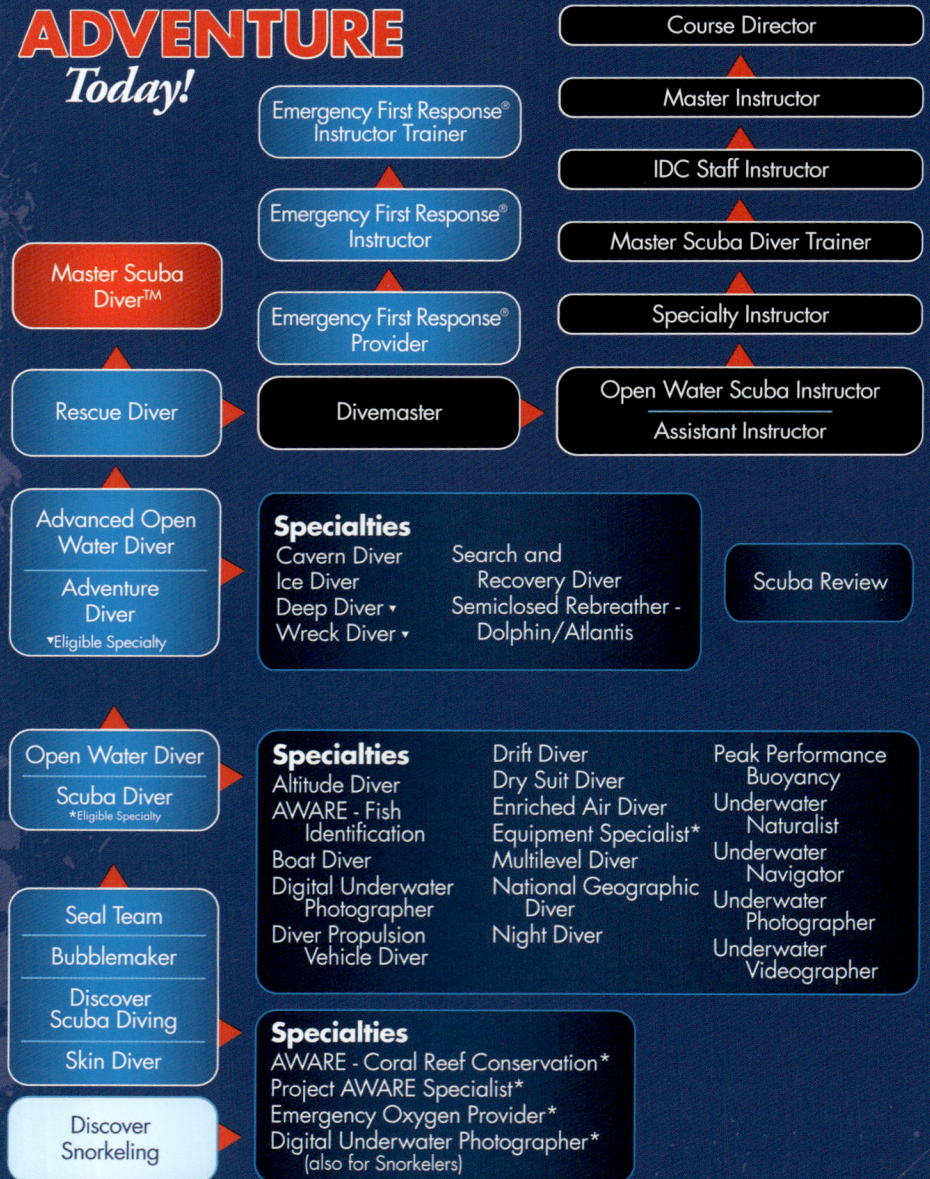

Course Director

↑

Master Instructor

↑

IDC Staff Instructor

↑

Master Scuba Diver Trainer

↑

Specialty Instructor

↑

Open Water Scuba Instructor / Assistant Instructor

Emergency First Response® Instructor Trainer

↑

Emergency First Response® Instructor

↑

Emergency First Response® Provider

Master Scuba Diver™

↑

Rescue Diver → Divemaster →

↑

Advanced Open Water Diver / Adventure Diver
▾Eligible Specialty

Specialties
Cavern Diver
Ice Diver
Deep Diver ▾
Wreck Diver ▾
Search and Recovery Diver
Semiclosed Rebreather - Dolphin/Atlantis

Scuba Review

↑

Open Water Diver / Scuba Diver
*Eligible Specialty

Specialties
Altitude Diver
AWARE - Fish Identification
Boat Diver
Digital Underwater Photographer
Diver Propulsion Vehicle Diver
Drift Diver
Dry Suit Diver
Enriched Air Diver
Equipment Specialist*
Multilevel Diver
National Geographic Diver
Night Diver
Peak Performance Buoyancy
Underwater Naturalist
Underwater Navigator
Underwater Photographer
Underwater Videographer

↑

Seal Team
Bubblemaker
Discover Scuba Diving
Skin Diver

Specialties
AWARE - Coral Reef Conservation*
Project AWARE Specialist*
Emergency Oxygen Provider*
Digital Underwater Photographer*
(also for Snorkelers)

Discover Snorkeling →

*For all level of diver or non-diver.

Why Divers Dive with *Enriched Air*

Advantages and Disadvantages of Diving with Enriched Air and Enriched Air Computers

Study Objectives

Underline/highlight the answers to these questions as you read:

1. What is "enriched air"?

2. What is the primary benefit of using enriched air?

3. How does using enriched air affect no stop limits?

4. Why is it too simplistic to say enriched air is safer than air when diving well within air no decompression limits?

5. How does using enriched air affect narcosis when diving?

6. What are three advantages of using an enriched air dive computer for enriched air diving?

What's Enriched Air?

Although enriched air nitrox is common and popularly used in recreational diving, you may not know exactly what it is. You may recall from your PADI Open Water Diver course that air consists of approximately 79% nitrogen and 21% oxygen. *Enriched air* has been enriched with oxygen (had oxygen added), so it has more than 21% oxygen. Enriched air is any nitrogen/oxygen gas blend with more than 21% oxygen.

As you'll see shortly, the purpose isn't to have more oxygen but to have a lower proportion of nitrogen. But, much of what you'll learn in this course relates to the higher percentage of oxygen in your breathing gas.

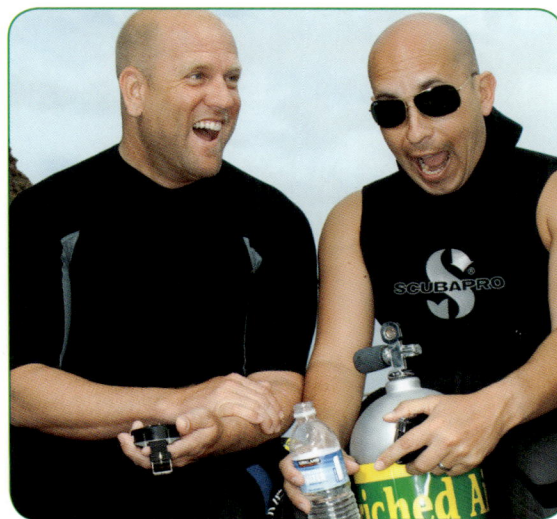

You may have also noticed that there are several names divers commonly use when talking about enriched air nitrox. These include "EANx" and "EAN" (from **E**nriched **A**ir **N**itrox), "nitrox" and "enriched air." All of these mean the same thing (although "nitrox" actually includes nitrogen/oxygen blends with a *lower* oxygen percentage than air has), and you'll see and hear them all in this course just as you will when diving. When referring to a specific nitrox blend, it's common to write "EANx" followed by its oxygen percentage. For example, EANx36 is nitrox with 36% oxygen. You would say "EANx36," "Enriched Air 36," "Enriched Air Nitrox 36" or "Nitrox 36."

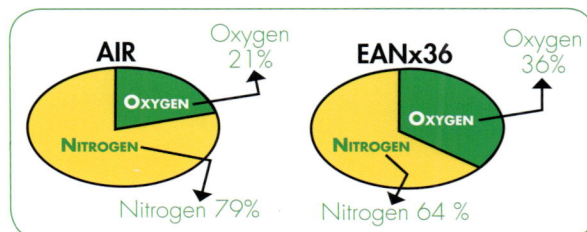

Air consists of approximately 79% nitrogen and 21% oxygen. Enriched air has more oxygen and less nitrogen. EANx36, for example, consists of approximately 64% nitrogen and 36% oxygen.

3

Why Use It?

The primary benefit of using enriched air nitrox is that it exposes you to less nitrogen than when you dive with air. This provides some advantages:

- It extends your allowable bottom time.

- It reduces any need to "push" (near) the air no decompression limits.

- It reduces your overall nitrogen load on multiple dives.

The higher the oxygen content of the EANx blend, the less nitrogen you breathe. Within limits, your body metabolizes or otherwise absorbs oxygen, so it doesn't contribute to bubble formation after a dive. This means that compared to air, for a given dive you absorb less nitrogen. This allows longer no decompression limits. How much longer depends upon the oxygen percentage, but here are some examples.

Depth	Air No D limit	EANx32 No D limit	EANx36 No D limit
18 metres	56 min	95 min	125 min
22 metres	37 min	60 min	70 min
50 feet	80 min	155 min	220 min
80 feet	30 min	45 min	55 min

The amount of added no stop time compared to air is even longer when you combine enriched air with an enriched air computer. This is because you benefit from the extended dive times that result from both lower nitrogen absorption and from slower absorption when you ascend to a shallower depth on a multilevel profile.

The advantage of enriched air becomes especially evident when you make two or more dives because you have less residual nitrogen reducing your repetitive dive times. Using enriched air and an enriched air dive computer, depending upon depth, you'll commonly find that it's the quantity of enriched air you have in your cylinder that limits you, not the no stop limits. It's common to note this particularly when making several dives daily over the course of a multiple day dive trip.

Enriched Air and Safety

Since the early 1990s, recreational divers have made hundreds of thousands of enriched air dives successfully. Through these data and this field experience, the enriched air no decompression limits and concepts have established themselves as being as reliable as those of normal air. Using enriched air dive computers has become commonplace, and statistics indicate that the DCI rate for diving with EANx is essentially the same as for air diving.

Although you reduce your nitrogen exposure with enriched air, keep in mind that you increase your oxygen exposure. Oxygen has its own set of potential problems, some of which, if disregarded, can be significantly more hazardous than problems associated with nitrogen. In this course, you learn the procedures and guidelines that keep your oxygen exposure within accepted limits. They're neither complex nor difficult – but they are important.

Logically, if you make a given dive breathing enriched air, you finish with less dissolved nitrogen in your body than if you had made the same dive using normal air. This is a good thing, however it would be too simplistic to state that when well within air limits, enriched air is "safer" than air. As you will see, higher oxygen levels create a potential hazard that hardly exist in air diving within recreational limits.

You certainly can choose to use enriched air to reduce your nitrogen exposure by following an air computer while actually breathing enriched air. This may be attractive if you are subject to one or more of the factors that make decompression sickness (DCS) more likely.

For example, based on the Recreational Dive Planner, a non multilevel dive to 18 metres/60 feet for 55 minutes with air is a no stop dive that pushes the limits — not a recommended practice. The same dive with EANx32 would be well within limits. For such dives, using EANx may be a better choice, even though it's technically possible to use air.

A second point is that the DCI incidence rate is already very low in recreational air diving. Simply switching to EANx would not be expected to change the rate significantly. Whether you have enriched air available or not, you should always apply other steps that tangibly reduce risk. These include making safety stops, maintaining a proper ascent rate and avoiding predisposing DCS factors such as dehydration, smoking or excessive alcohol consumption. These are still sensible precautions to take routinely even though you are now able to use enriched air.

Enriched Air and Narcosis

Nitrogen narcosis is a well known problem for divers and it used to be assumed that breathing less nitrogen would reduce its effects. Although enriched air reduces the amount of nitrogen you breathe underwater, many diving physiologists believe it does not significantly reduce narcosis. This is because, theoretically, oxygen has about the same narcotic potential as nitrogen. Further, studies have found little difference between the narcotic effects

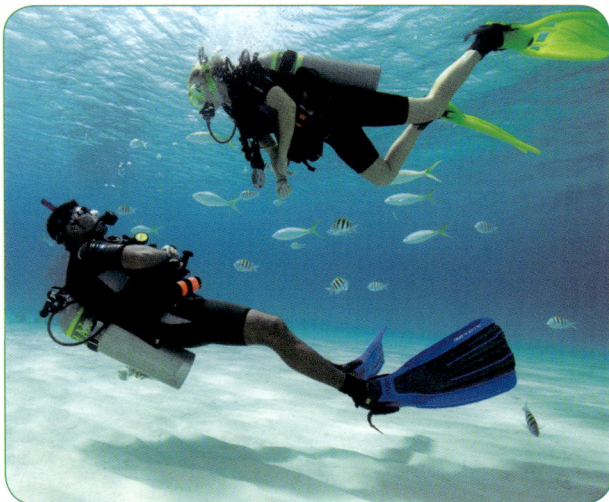

There's no meaningful difference in narcosis between enriched air nitrox and air. Plan EANx dives accounting for narcosis just as you would with air.

of nitrogen and oxygen. So, while enriched air has less nitrogen, the current thinking is the narcosis potential is the same. This means you should plan an enriched air dive accounting for narcosis just as you would using air.

Keep in mind that divers' susceptibility to narcosis differs, and susceptibility may change from one dive to the next. You may feel no narcosis on one dive at a certain depth, but feel its effects on another dive to the same depth. There are some other factors like fatigue, exertion, or task loading that may influence the effects of narcosis.

The Physiology of Diving in *The Encyclopedia of Recreational Diving*

Learn more...

Advantages of Using an Enriched Air Dive Computer

Today most divers use dive computers when they dive enriched air nitrox to benefit from three primary advantages.

The first, as discussed above, is that computers combine enriched air with multilevel diving for the most no stop time possible. You really see the difference in added no stop dive time when making two or more repetitive dives.

Second, most models will or can be set to alert you if you accidentally exceed the maximum depth for your gas blend. As a certified diver, you know that you should always watch your depth, but exceeding your planned depth can be serious with EANx (more about maximum limits shortly). The ability for the computer to alert you to take corrective action is a significant secondary benefit.

Third, dive computers simplify diving planning and execution by calculating both your oxygen exposure and your allowable no stop time, and warn you if you near the limits of either. You can do this with tables, but while it's not difficult, it does add several steps to calculating dive limits and dive planning. Enriched air dive computers are much more convenient.

Diving nitrox with an enriched air dive computer maximizes your no stop dive time, provides maximum depth alerts and is more convenient.

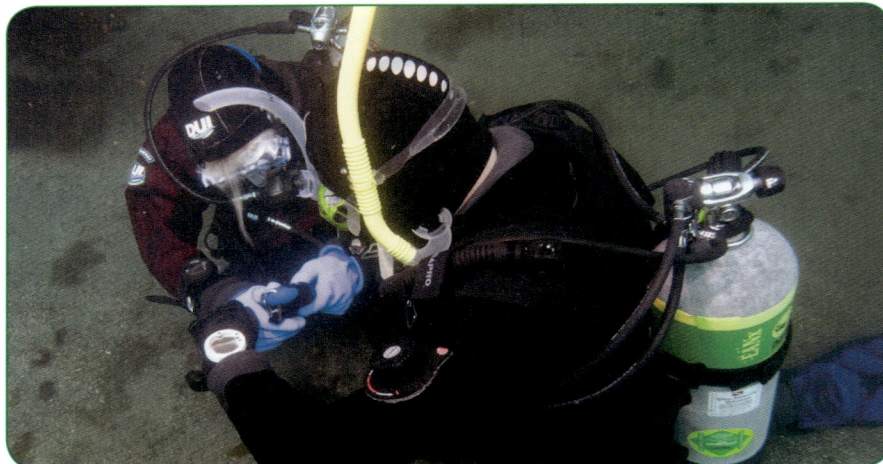

Exercise 1

1. "Enriched air" is

   ☐ a. any mixture of oxygen and nitrogen.
   ☐ b. a mixture of oxygen and nitrogen with more than 21% oxygen.
   ☐ c. air enriched with helium.

2. The primary benefit of using enriched air is that it lets you

   ☐ a. dive deeper.
   ☐ b. dive longer.

3. Enriched air _____ the no stop limits compared to air.

   ☐ a. extends
   ☐ b. reduces
   ☐ c. does nothing to

4. It is too simplistic to say enriched air is safer than air when well within air no stop limits because enriched air creates an oxygen hazard and the DCI rate is already very low in recreational air diving.

   ☐ True   ☐ False

5. Using enriched air _____ narcosis when diving.

   ☐ a. reduces
   ☐ b. increases
   ☐ c. has no effect on

6. Advantages of using an enriched air dive computer for enriched air diving include (check all that apply):

   ☐ a. providing maximum no stop time by combining EANx and multilevel diving.
   ☐ b. the ability to warn you if you exceed your maximum depth.
   ☐ c. simplifying dive planning.

How did you do?

1. *b.* 2. *b.* 3. *a.* 4. *True.* 5. *c.* 6. *a, b, c.*

Gear and *Stuff*

Enriched Air Equipment Considerations

Study Objectives

Underline/highlight the answers to these questions as you read:

1. What is the primary concern regarding enriched air and scuba equipment?

2. What are the requirements and recommendations for scuba equipment (other than cylinders) used with enriched air with up to 40 percent oxygen?

3. Why does enriched air diving require a dedicated cylinder?

4. What color coding, stickers (decals) and tags should an enriched air cylinder have?

5. What are the two primary concerns associated with filling enriched air cylinders, and how are they avoided?

6. Why should only qualified, reputable enriched air blenders fill enriched air cylinders?

7. What is the potential hazard of improper enriched air filling procedures?

8. What should you do if an enriched air cylinder or oxygen-serviced equipment is used with standard compressed air?

9. How do you identify qualified enriched air blenders and enriched air service?

10. What are the two most commonly used *blends of enriched air*?

Requirements and Recommendations

The primary concern regarding enriched air and your dive equipment is the high oxygen content. Some materials

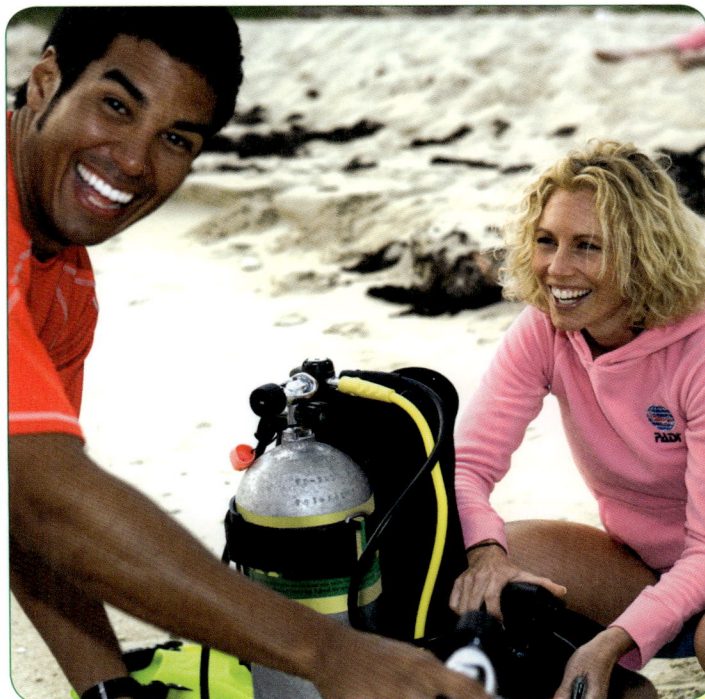

burn or explode readily when in contact with high oxygen gas blends (or pure oxygen), even at normal room temperature. Exposure to high oxygen gas blends may also cause some types of equipment material to deteriorate rapidly.

These problems arise because fire, explosion and deterioration are forms of *oxidation* – a chemical reaction involving oxygen. The more oxygen in contact with a material, the more readily oxidation can occur. To address this, the following guidelines apply to all scuba equipment *except* the cylinder:

1. The common dive community guideline is that scuba regulators, BCDs, SPGs and alternate air sources may be used with enriched air blends that have up to 40% oxygen without modification. This guideline, originally based on the standards and field experience of NOAA, the US Navy, the US Occupational Safety and Health Administration (OSHA) and others, has

been in use for more than a decade with a good record.

2. Gas mixes with more than 40% oxygen require equipment (including cylinders) that has been cleaned to *oxygen service specifications*. This means the equipment must be specially cleaned, be made of oxygen compatible materials and be lubricated with oxygen compatible lubricants. Blends with more than 40% oxygen are uncommon in recreational diving, and are generally used when diving with recreational semiclosed circuit rebreathers.

3. Some scuba manufacturers state that their equipment shouldn't be used with enriched air. Others state that their equipment may be used with enriched air, but that it requires special servicing and maintenance. Follow all manufacturer recommendations with respect to using equipment with enriched air.

4. The use of oxygen compatible lubricants, O-rings and other materials as appropriate during servicing is generally recommended.

5. You should have your regulator serviced at least annually (or as stipulated by the manufacturer), preferably by a scuba technician qualified to work on enriched air equipment. If your equipment is accidentally exposed to anything other than water (i.e., oils, lubricants not recommended by the manufacturer, etc.), have it inspected or recleaned by a qualified technician to ensure that it hasn't picked up anything incompatible for use with enriched air. If you add any accessories, such as low pressure hoses, follow manufacturer recommendations.

Local law or standards may require that all equipment used with enriched air be cleaned to oxygen service specifications. Local practice may also require that specific equipment meets oxygen service standards. For

example, enriched air cylinders and regulators rated for 300 bar/4400 psi are often oxygen service rated. In some areas, such as Europe, the standard requires a special valve and regulator for enriched air equipment (M26x2).

The recommendations for equipment used with enriched air may change. Stay informed and follow current manufacturer recommendations for your equipment.

Cylinders Used for Enriched Air Diving

Even when you can use the regulator you already have for enriched air nitrox with up to 40% oxygen (depending upon the make, model and local regulations), you will need a dedicated cylinder (scuba tank). There are two reasons:

First, it's important that no one accidentally confuse an enriched air cylinder for a one of normal air. Enriched air cylinders are clearly marked.

Second, one common method for blending enriched air requires putting pure oxygen in the cylinder and then adding oxygen compatible air. This is called *partial pressure blending*. **Because the cylinder valve and interior will be in contact with pure oxygen, if partial pressure blending with oxygen will be used, the cylinder must meet oxygen service standards, even if the final enriched air blend will have less than 40% oxygen.** This means that besides being marked properly, cylinders used for partial pressure blending must be cleaned and lubricated for oxygen exposure, and all O-rings, gaskets and other valve materials must be oxygen compatible. **The standard scuba cylinder doesn't meet these requirements.**

Enriched air cylinders filled by other blending methods (premix/membrane methods) may not have to meet oxygen service standards, depending upon manufacturer recommendations, local law or local practice, but the cylinder must still be dedicated and have the proper markings.

Enriched Air Cylinder Markings

Enriched air cylinders have standardized stickers and/or tags and color coding generally agreed upon and accepted by the broad international dive community. These markings assure that you can readily identify an enriched air cylinder, that you can determine its contents and that you can tell whether the cylinder can be used for partial pressure blending:

1. Yellow cylinders should have a 10 centimetre/4 inch green band around the shoulder with yellow or white lettering reading "Enriched Air," "Enriched Air Nitrox," "Nitrox" or a similar designation.

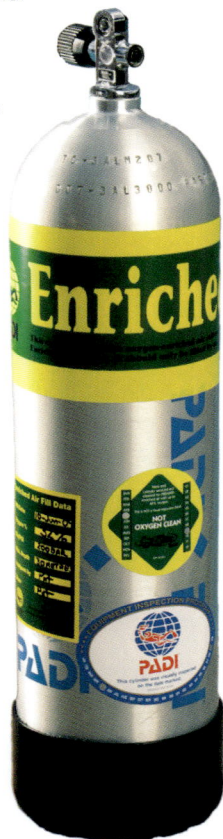

2. Non-yellow cylinders should have a 15 centimetre/6 inch band around the shoulder. The top and bottom of this band should be a yellow, 2.5 cm/1 in. band, with the center 10 cm/4 in. of green. The green portion should have yellow or white lettering reading "Enriched Air," "Enriched Air Nitrox," "Nitrox" or a similar designation.

Non-yellow cylinders should have a band around the tank shoulder. The top and bottom should be yellow, with the center green. The green portion should have yellow or white lettering reading "Enriched Air," "Enriched Air Nitrox," "Nitrox" or a similar designation.

3. Like any scuba cylinder, an enriched air cylinder should have a dated visual inspection sticker (decal) or stamp stating that the cylinder has been inspected for corrosion, stress, etc., for enriched air use. It should also have a sticker stating whether it does or does not meet oxygen service standards.

At one time it was common for a single sticker to serve as both the visual inspection sticker and an oxygen service sticker, and you may still see it on occasion. But, visual inspection and oxygen service are really two separate considerations, so the dive community has moved to using independent markings.

Besides a dated visual inspection sticker like you find on a standard scuba cylinder, an enriched air cylinder should also have a decal stating whether it does or does not meet oxygen service standards.

4. An enriched air cylinder should have a contents sticker (decal) or permanent tag. This sticker/tag should, at a minimum, list the oxygen content of the blend the cylinder currently holds, the fill date, the maximum depth for the blend and the name of the person who analyzed the oxygen content to verify the blender's analysis (this should be the diver who will use the cylinder). Stickers are replaced and tags rewritten when you have the cylinder refilled. Do not remove the sticker or erase the tag after using the cylinder (the blender will do this when

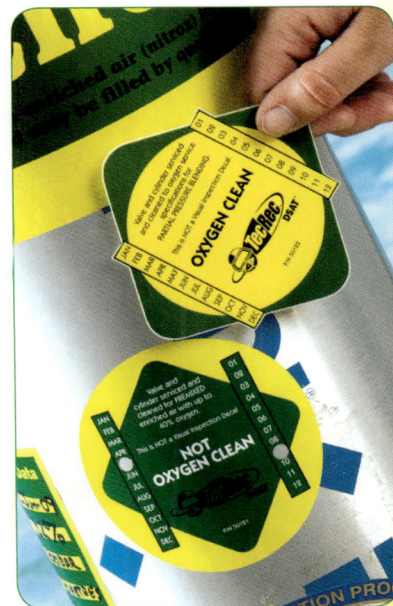

refilling the cylinder). If a permanent tag is used, the cylinder's serial number should be on the tag to prevent it from accidentally getting switched to another cylinder.

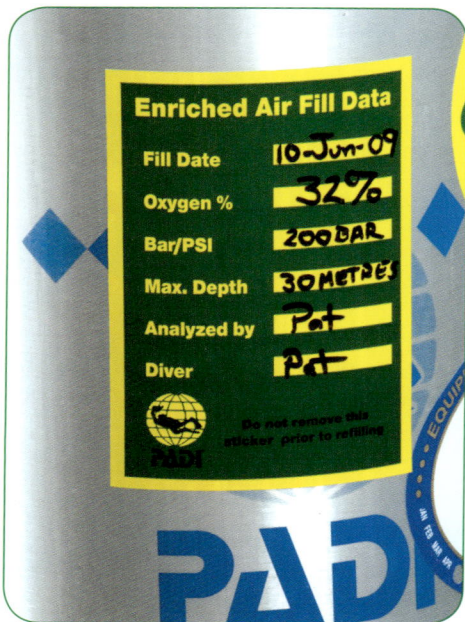

An enriched air cylinder should have a contents sticker (decal) or permanent tag. This sticker/tag should, at a minimum, list the oxygen content of the blend the cylinder currently holds, the fill date, the maximum depth for the blend and the name of the person who analyzed the oxygen content to verify the blender's analysis.

5. Although these are the broadly accepted markings, in some areas local laws, regulations and standards set differing or additional requirements. For example, in Europe, EANx cylinders have a white shoulder with a black stripe, and generally the entire cylinder is white. Some areas have recommendations or requirements that an enriched air cylinder be used within a given period, such as within 30 days of filling, and the cylinder may be marked accordingly. In other areas, the practice is

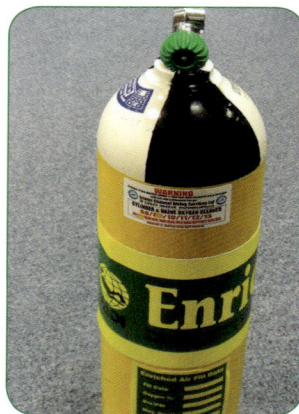

In the UK, for example, EANx cylinders are required to have the black and white shoulder pattern shown. Many UK dive operations use the international community standard markings, as well, as shown.

to mark regular cylinders "Air Only," which helps further differentiate them from EANx cylinders. Your instructor will tell you about any that apply to your local area.

Filling Enriched Air Cylinders

There are two concerns with filling enriched air cylinders that you don't have when filling a normal air cylinder. Again, both of these concerns arise from the high oxygen content of enriched air.

1. Fire/explosion hazard. You've already learned that many substances readily burn or explode when in contact with pure oxygen or high proportions of oxygen. These substances include trace hydrocarbons (lubricants) found in normal compressed scuba air. Trace lubricants accumulate over time in a standard air cylinder. This creates a hazard immediately if oxygen were put into the cylinder. Therefore, normal compressed air can create a hazard if it comes in contact with high oxygen concentrations. This is why blenders use *oxygen compatible air* for partial pressure blending.

This concern is greatest when partial pressure filling will be used, since the cylinder and system may be exposed to pure oxygen. Filling systems that don't require putting oxygen into the scuba cylinder minimize these risks. These include membrane systems, which do not use pure oxygen at all, and premixing enriched air in large storage cylinders that the blender can readily protect from contaminants.

⚠️ **Never have an enriched air cylinder filled by a station that does not handle enriched air. Enriched air should never be put into a cylinder that is not dedicated to EANx.**

Always have an enriched air cylinder filled only by a qualified enriched air blender, even if you want only air in it (more about this shortly). This effectively manages the biggest concern regarding oxygen compatibility and enriched air scuba cylinders.

2. **Percentage of oxygen in the blend.** The other concern with enriched air fills is oxygen content. The amount of oxygen in an enriched air blend affects your no stop time and oxygen exposure. If the content changes by more than 1%, your maximum allowable depth and no decompression limits will change. Your computer will adjust for these changes, but having more oxygen or less oxygen than you asked for may restrict the maximum depth or no stop dive time, respectively, that you planned on having.

To manage these concerns, enriched air blenders are trained to follow strict guidelines with procedures and special equipment that aren't needed for air fills. To begin, enriched air fill stations will only fill a properly designated enriched air cylinder.

If the station uses partial pressure blending, the blender checks whether the cylinder is marked as cleaned to oxygen compatible standards. If not, the blender will only use a system that does not expose it to more than 40% oxygen. During blending with oxygen, the station uses oxygen compatible air that is produced by using special oil free compressors, special filtration or a combination of both. *This is crucial because even trace amounts of oil or contaminants may create a fire/ explosion hazard.*

Because of the potential hazards of partial pressure blending with pure oxygen in the scuba cylinder, more and more enriched air fill stations are switching to alternative methods for blending enriched air. These methods include special membranes that separate oxygen from nitrogen during filling, and constant flow blending that adds a small amount of oxygen before compression. Other centers purchase premixed enriched air from industrial gas companies, and some partial pressure blend only in their own bank cylinders. With all of these methods, your cylinder will be filled with preblended enriched air, reducing the potential for fire/ explosion hazard.

Enriched air blending procedures also assure accurate blending. After blending, as a double check the blender analyzes the enriched air to assure it has the intended percentage of oxygen, then records the analysis and other information in a permanent log. Before diving with an enriched air cylinder, you need to personally reconfirm the blender's analysis. (More about this later.)

Again, you easily handle enriched air fill concerns by having only reputable, qualified enriched air blenders fill enriched air cylinders for you.

⚠️ **Attempting to blend enriched air without following proper filling procedures can be very hazardous. Never put pure oxygen in a standard cylinder and fill it or have it filled from a conventional scuba air fill station in an attempt to make enriched air. This practice poses a high risk of fire or explosion.**

If you ever need to use air in an enriched air cylinder, no problem: Take it to an enriched air fill center. They treat the fill as enriched air in all respects, including marking it EANx21 ("enriched" air with 21% oxygen), analyzing the contents and completing all records. If an enriched air cylinder that has been prepared for

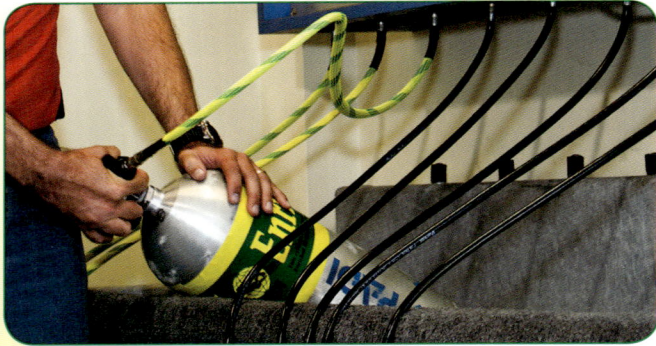

To address concerns related to safely handling high oxygen percentages and obtaining accurate blends, enriched air blenders follow strict guidelines and procedures that aren't needed for regular air fills.

Local Variations

Some countries, including several in Europe, require a special dedicated enriched air nitrox valve on enriched air cylinders (M26x2). In this case, your regulator requires a compatible fitting. Your instructor will advise you if this applies in the area where you're taking this course.

oxygen service (for partial pressure filling) is accidentally filled from a conventional air source, **it must be serviced and cleaned by someone qualified to service enriched air equipment** before being exposed to more than 40% oxygen again. Some manufacturers have similar recommendations for other equipment specially modified or serviced for use with enriched air.

The Mix Masters: Enriched Air Blenders

You can identify qualified enriched air blenders and enriched air service by looking for the following:

- Gas quality verification — The operation should be able to show regular analysis of the air it uses for enriched air blending. This air should meet local standards for oxygen compatible air.

- Proper procedures, cylinder markings, analysis and record keeping — A lack of these may indicate that the operation isn't qualified or prepared to properly support enriched air diving.

- Documentation — The operation and/or individuals working there should be able to show evidence of training and certification as DSAT Gas Blenders (or other blender certification). You may look for records from private organizations such as ASTM (American Society for Testing and Materials) the Compressed Gas Association, a government agency such as NOAA or other recognized public or private bodies.

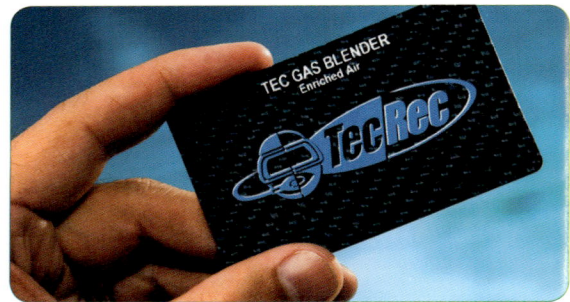

Reputable EANx blenders have documentation showing their qualifications for producing enriched air, such as the Tec Gas Blender certification.

Two Most Common Blends

Although the PADI Enriched Air Diver course qualifies you to use a range of enriched air blends, there are two that you'll probably use often because they're commonly available:

1. EANx32, also known as "NOAA Nitrox I"

and

2. EANx36, also known as "NOAA Nitrox II."

These blends were first put into common use by NOAA and many enriched air stations store them premixed. Because of their utility, these blends are by far the most popular with recreational divers. At some enriched air stations you may have to wait for any other blend. Some supply *only* EANx32 and EANx36.

Exercise 2

1. The primary concern regarding enriched air and scuba equipment is:

   ☐ a. that improper equipment will affect the percentage of oxygen breathed.

   ☐ b. that contact with high oxygen content may cause fire, explosion or deterioration.

   ☐ c. that your dive buddy may not know what blend you're using.

   ☐ d. that local regulations may prohibit enriched air equipment.

2. When using enriched air with up to 40% oxygen (check all that apply):

   ☐ a. Generally, you may use standard scuba equipment (except cylinder).

   ☐ b. You may use standard scuba equipment including cylinder.

   ☐ c. Use of oxygen compatible lubricants is generally recommended.

   ☐ d. Follow all manufacturer recommendations regarding using their equipment with enriched air.

3. Enriched air requires a dedicated cylinder because (check all that apply):

   ☐ a. it can be hazardous to unknowingly dive with enriched air.

   ☐ b. it can be hazardous to blend enriched air in a conventional air cylinder.

   ☐ c. enriched air cylinders have special considerations when transported by truck.

   ☐ d. enriched air cylinders have a shorter expected use cycle than air cylinders.

4. Based on broadly accepted international dive community practices, enriched air cylinders should have the following markings/colors/tags (check all that apply):

   ☐ a. Yellow cylinders should have a 10 cm/4 in green band at the shoulder with "Enriched Air," "Enriched Air Nitrox," "Nitrox" or a similar designation.

   ☐ b. The cylinder should have a standard visual inspection sticker.

   ☐ c. The cylinder should have a contents sticker (decal) or tag.

   ☐ d. The cylinder should have sticker (decal) to indicate whether it is oxygen service rated.

5. The two primary concerns associated with filling enriched air cylinders are fire/explosion hazards and accurate filling. These are managed by having your cylinder filled by qualified enriched air blenders, who use proper procedures for filling and gas analysis.

   ☐ True   ☐ False

6. Only qualified, reputable enriched air blenders should fill enriched air cylinders because they have the training and equipment to minimize the problems associated with filling enriched air cylinders.

   ☐ True   ☐ False

7. The potential hazards that can arise from filling an enriched air cylinder improperly include (check all that apply):

   ☐ a. Fire   ☐ c. Decompression illness
   ☐ b. Explosion   ☐ d. Oxygen toxicity

8. If an oxygen service rated enriched air cylinder is filled with standard compressed air, you should:

   ☐ a. refill it with enriched air very cautiously.

   ☐ b. have it serviced by someone qualified to work on enriched air equipment.

   ☐ c. destroy the cylinder.

   ☐ d. No special action is required.

9. In looking for qualified enriched air service, look for (check all that apply):

   ☐ a. Gas quality verification.

   ☐ b. Green scuba tanks.

   ☐ c. Proper enriched air procedures.

   ☐ d. Blender certification such as Tec Gas Blender.

10. The two most common blends of enriched air are:

    ☐ a. EANx30 and EANx40
    ☐ b. EANx30 and EANx36
    ☐ c. EANx32 and EANx40
    ☐ d. EANx32 and EANx36

How did you do?

1. *b.* 2. *a, c, d. b is incorrect because EANx always requires a dedicated cylinder.* 3. *a, b.* 4. *a, b, c, d.* 5. *True.* 6. *True.* 7. *a, b.* 8. *b.* 9. *a, c, d. b is incorrect because green cylinders do not indicate an enriched air fill source.* 10. *d.*

Oxygen *Exposure*

Prevention and Management

Study Objectives

Underline/highlight the answers to these questions as you read:

1. What is meant by oxygen partial pressure?

2. How does exposure to increased oxygen partial pressure affect allowable dive time?

3. What are the maximum and contingency oxygen partial pressure limits?

4. What is the primary hazard of exceeding the oxygen exposure limits?

5. What six signs and symptoms may precede a convulsion caused by oxygen toxicity?

6. What should you do if you experience any symptoms of oxygen toxicity?

7. How do you use an EANx compatible dive computer to manage oxygen exposure and remain within accepted limits?

8. What should you do if you accidentally exceed the oxygen exposure limits for your computer?

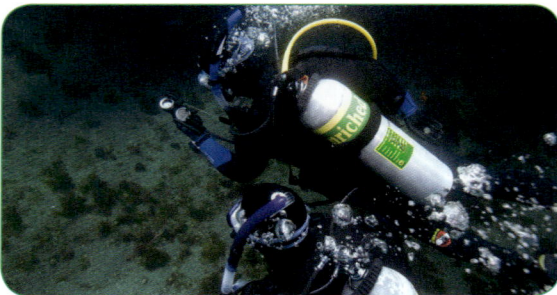

Oxygen Partial Pressure

When diving with air within recreational diving limits, oxygen exposure is not an issue. Due to the high oxygen content, however, oxygen exposure can be an issue when diving with EANx. As an Enriched Air Diver, you will use your dive computer to manage your oxygen exposure to keep it within accepted limits.

To avoid oxygen toxicity, you measure the oxygen concentration you're breathing based on the oxygen percentage and your depth. Generally, oxygen concentration is measured as *oxygen partial pressure*.

Oxygen partial pressure refers to the pressure exerted only by the oxygen part of the blend, hence the name "partial" pressure – it is only part of the total pressure. In diving, partial pressure is usually expressed in "atmospheres," and abbreviated "ata" for "atmospheres absolute." Regions using the metric system use absolute bar, which, while technically slightly different from an atmosphere, are commonly used interchangeably in a diving context. You can use the terms interchangeably with respect to this course. Oxygen partial pressure is sometimes abbreviated "PO_2" or "O_2 p.p.," so you might see a reference to "PO_2 0.21 ata," for example, or "PO_2 0.21 bar." The convention is so strong that often divers drop the ata/bar reference entirely: "PO_2 0.21," with the atmospheres/ bar understood.

An atmosphere or bar, as you may recall from your Open Water Diver course, is pressure equal to the air pressure surrounding us at sea level. Underwater, the total pressure increases one atmosphere/bar for each 10 metres/33 feet of seawater we descend. Mathematically, the oxygen partial pressure is simply the percentage of oxygen in the enriched air times the pressure at depth in ata/bar.

For example, if you dive to 10 metres/33 feet using EANx40, what would the oxygen partial pressure be? At 10 metres/33 feet, the pressure is two atmospheres/ bar – one of water and one of air. The enriched air has 40% oxygen, so 2 ata/bar x .40 = .80 ata/bar oxygen partial pressure. (Remember that with percentages, you move the decimal two places to the left before multiplying, adding, dividing, etc., with another number, so that "40%" is ".40," and "5%" is ".05," etc.)

Partial Pressure Comparison			
Depth	Pressure	PO_2 Using Air	PO_2 Using EANx40
0	1 ata/bar	.21 ata/bar	.4 ata/bar
10m/33ft	2 ata/bar	.42 ata/bar	.8 ata/bar
20m/66ft	3 ata/bar	.63 ata/bar	1.2 ata/bar

The greater the oxygen percent and/or the deeper you dive, the higher the oxygen partial pressure. Don't worry – you're not going to be doing a lot of math here. Your EANx dive computer does this for you. But, you need to understand what oxygen partial pressures are and how they're calculated because they're the basis for determining oxygen exposure limits.

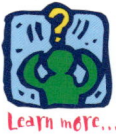

The Physics of Diving in *The Encyclopedia of Recreational Diving*

Learn more...

Oxygen Exposure Limits

The higher oxygen partial pressures you experience with enriched air nitrox must be kept within limits to avoid oxygen toxicity, which can be a serious hazard. This means that exposure to increased oxygen partial pressure decreases your allowable dive time.

Your EANx dive computer tracks your oxygen exposure much as it does your exposure to nitrogen, and it's important to stay well within the limits, just as it is with nitrogen (in recreational diving with nitrox, it's still *usually* your no stop time, not oxygen exposure, that limits your allowable dive time.)

Oxygen exposure limits relate entirely to the oxygen partial pressure. In the previous example, the oxygen partial pressure is .80 ata at 10 metres/33 feet using EANx40. If you were to dive with EANx36, you would have the same partial pressure at 12 metres/40 feet. Your oxygen exposure limits are the same for either dive, and your dive computer would show the same oxygen exposure limits.

Besides oxygen exposure over time, there are *oxygen partial pressure limits* that you must stay within *regardless of time*. **The maximum oxygen partial pressure limit for enriched air diving is 1.4 ata/bar.** You will learn to plan your dives so that you don't exceed the depth at which the blend you're using reaches 1.4. Planning your dive to reach less than 1.4 gives you some margin for error.

In addition to managing your oxygen exposure, another reason 1.4 ata/bar makes an effective maximum limit is that oxygen may contribute to bubble formation at higher partial pressures. While this is theoretical, staying within 1.4 ata/bar reduces the likelihood of any problems that may exist.

Some individuals retain carbon dioxide, which is thought to contribute to oxygen toxicity. Some tests show that a 1.4 ata/bar limit reduces oxygen toxicity risk for those few individuals who retain carbon dioxide. [1]*If your planned dive would exceed 1.4, select an enriched air with less oxygen, plan a shallower dive, or both.*

The *contingency* oxygen partial pressure limit is 1.6 ata/bar. Dives beyond this limit have the potential for immediate oxygen toxicity.

Consider the contingency limit – the partial pressures between 1.4 and 1.6 ata/bar – a margin for error only. You'll find that dive computers and tables often

[1]* D. Kerem, Y.I. Daskalovic, R. Arieli & A. Shupak, CO2 retention during hyperbaric exercise while breathing 40/60 nitrox, Undersea & Hyperbaric Medicine, Dec. 1995

provide oxygen exposure information for these partial pressures, but this is for emergency planning purposes only – something you use only if you accidentally

⚠️ exceed 1.4, creating a contingency situation. Divers have had oxygen toxicity while breathing oxygen partial pressures at or near 1.6 ata/bar.

Set your computer so the maximum oxygen partial pressure it allows is 1.4 ata/bar. Most computers will let you do this, or are preset for this limit. Once it's set, with most models it stays set unless you change it. Almost all models alert you with visual and/or audible signals if you exceed the limit you set. Some computers display your current PO_2 throughout the dive, whereas others only alert you if you exceed the maximum. Your instructor and/or the manufacturer literature can give you specifics on the settings and warnings for your specific computer.

⚠️ Exceeding accepted oxygen limits poses a high risk of oxygen toxicity. That's a strong but important statement, though it's not difficult to stay within accepted limits. If you were to exceed the contingency depth limit of 1.6 ata/bar for a blend accidentally, immediately ascend above the maximum depth (1.4 ata/bar) and end the dive.

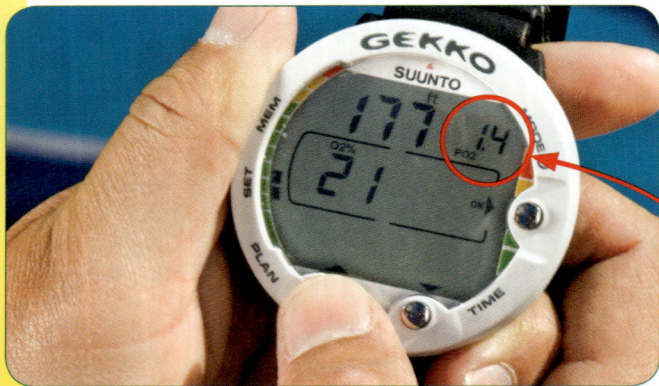

Set your enriched air dive computer so the maximum oxygen partial pressure it allows is 1.4 ata. Some come preset for this limit.

Do not make a repetitive dive, and follow your dive computer's instructions.

Oxygen Toxicity

CNS Toxicity

There are two types of oxygen toxicity that can occur

⚠️ by exceeding oxygen limits. **The primary hazard of exceeding the oxygen exposure limits is a fatal accident due to convulsing and drowning.** This can happen due to *central nervous system* (CNS) toxicity. CNS toxicity may cause a diver to convulse. Convulsions are not usually harmful in themselves, but underwater the diver is almost certain to lose the regulator and drown.

Therefore, it is very important that you maintain good buoyancy control, navigate properly and pay attention to other factors, such as currents, that may affect your maximum depth.

Warning signs and symptoms may precede a CNS convulsion, but most of the time, CNS convulsions occur without warning. If signs and symptoms do occur, they don't appear instantly. Instead, they appear gradually and worsen over time.

The warning signs and symptoms for oxygen toxicity, if they do occur, include:

1. visual disturbances, including tunnel vision

2. ears ringing

3. nausea

4. twitching or muscle spasms, especially in the face

5. irritability, restlessness, euphoria or anxiety

6. dizziness

Some divers remember these by remembering VENTID — vision, ears, nausea, twitching, irritability and dizziness.

If you experience any CNS toxicity

⚠️ **symptoms, end the dive by beginning a normal ascent immediately.** There's no need for a rapid or panicked ascent – just start up immediately at a normal, safe rate. During a penetration dive (like cavern or wreck diving), ascending immediately may not be possible. Abort the dive and ascend as soon as possible. For recreational penetration dives, it's best to keep your oxygen partial pressure very low, or to simply use air.

Other factors may predispose divers to CNS toxicity. Heavy exercise is one of these. Avoid heavy exercise if you near or will near oxygen exposure limits. This is especially true if you accidentally exceed the depth at which oxygen partial pressure is 1.4 ata/bar or greater. Again, staying well within your computer limits gives you a margin for error and reduces risk.

Some drugs are CNS exciters believed to predispose you to CNS toxicity. As reported at the October 1995 American Academy of Underwater Sciences (AAUS) workshop on enriched air, this includes the decongestant Pseudoephedrine HCl (found in Sudafed™ and other decongestant products). It's generally recommended that divers avoid decongestants when diving anyway (because they may wear off during the dive, leading to a reverse block). If you're taking a prescription, be sure to consult with a physician knowledgeable in diving medicine before using the drug while diving (with air or enriched air).

As previously mentioned, carbon dioxide accumulation in the body may predispose you to oxygen toxicity. Breathe continuously (do not skip breathe) to avoid retaining carbon dioxide. It's quite rare for a diver who breathes normally to retain carbon dioxide, but if you frequently experience headaches after a dive, as a precaution, consult a physician familiar with diving to make sure you're not accumulating carbon dioxide while underwater.

It's important to keep oxygen exposure concerns and CNS toxicity in perspective. In recreational enriched air diving, you're far more likely to approach your nitrogen limits than any oxygen limit. By setting your dive computer properly and diving well within its limits, it's easy to manage oxygen concerns.

But, oxygen is an unforgiving gas and CNS oxygen toxicity underwater on scuba is usually fatal. Dive well within oxygen limits. Because people vary in their physiology, no dive table or computer can guarantee that oxygen toxicity will not occur, even within accepted limits.

In other words, while it's not hard to manage oxygen exposure risks, do not underestimate the consequences of failing to do so. Dive conservatively, well within all table, computer and maximum depth limits.

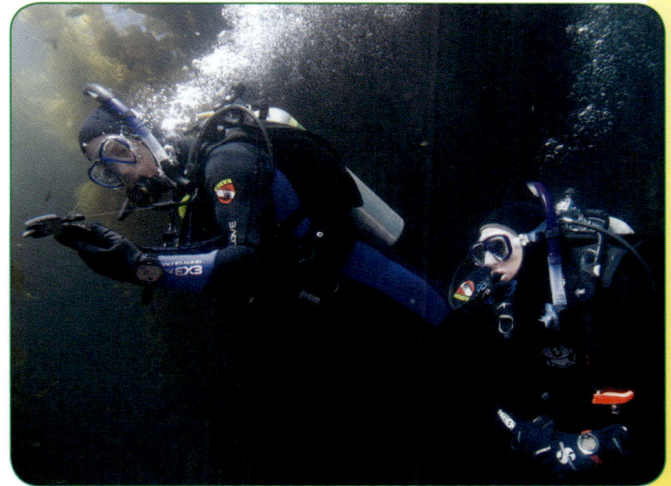

While it's not hard to manage oxygen exposure risks, do not underestimate the consequences of failing to do so. Dive conservatively, well within all table, computer and maximum depth limits.

Pulmonary Oxygen Toxicity

Another form of oxygen toxicity is *pulmonary* oxygen toxicity, which results from prolonged lung exposure to high oxygen partial pressures. This is *highly unlikely* within the oxygen limits of your computer while making no stop enriched air dives. This is mainly a concern for commercial or technical dives that require long decompression stops using pure or high amounts of oxygen (50% or more).

Nonetheless, you should be familiar with pulmonary toxicity because the possibility, while remote, does exist. The most common symptoms of pulmonary toxicity are irritation in the lungs, a burning sensation in the chest, coughing and reduction of the vital capacity (total amount of air you can inhale).

Typically, if it does occur and the diver discontinues diving before symptoms become severe, pulmonary toxicity clears up quickly and without complication given sufficient time at the surface breathing air. Still, in the unlikely event you experience any of the symptoms, as a precaution discontinue diving for a few days until the symptoms resolve, and consult a physician if symptoms are severe or prolonged.

The Physiology of Diving in *The Encyclopedia of Recreational Diving*

learn more...

Managing Oxygen Exposure

You use your enriched air compatible dive computer to help you manage your oxygen exposure so you stay well within limits.

The first step, as mentioned previously, is to set your dive computer for a maximum oxygen partial pressure of 1.4. See the manufacturer guidelines for doing this, and your instructor can help you. Once you have this set, most computers will remember this limit.

The second step is setting your computer for the specific enriched air blend you're using for your dive. This is essential so your computer can calculate both your no stop limits and your oxygen exposure. You'll learn more about this shortly.

Next, once your computer is set for your EANx blend, activate the scroll mode that shows your no stop limits. This is the same as when your computer's set for air, but you'll see longer time limits with EANx. Typically, your computer will give you depth and times in 3 metre/10 foot increments. With most models, the deepest depth displayed is the deepest depth you can reach without exceeding 1.4 ata/bar. (Some models display this based on 1.6 ata/bar, in which case use the table below to find the maximum depth.) Also, some

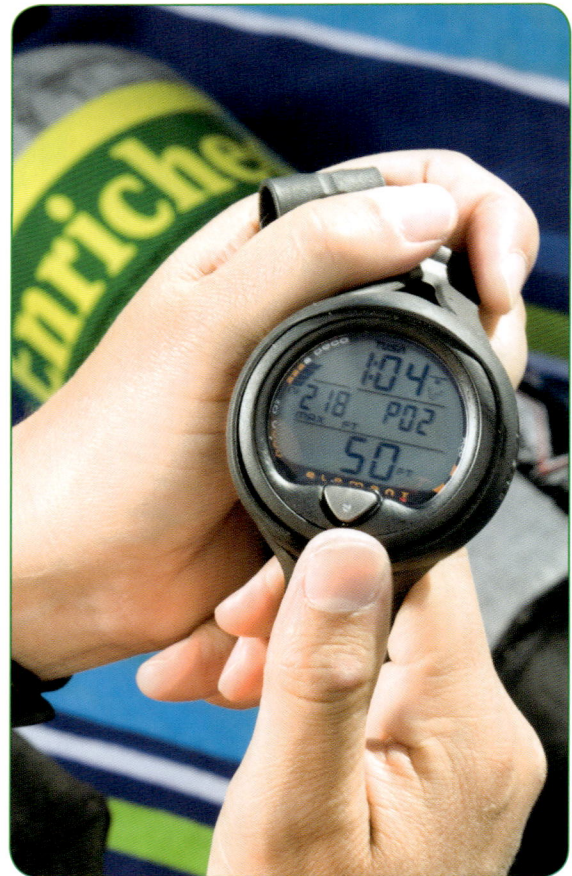

Once your computer's set for your EANx blend, activate the scroll mode that shows your no stop limits. With most models, the deepest depth displayed is the deepest depth you can reach without exceeding 1.4 ata/bar.

computers show you the maximum depth when you set the blend, and you don't have to use the scroll mode. (See the manufacturer's instructions for specifics for maximum and contingency depths with different blends.)

Regardless of how it's displayed, note this depth, because exceeding it would take your oxygen partial pressure above 1.4 and pose a serious risk of oxygen toxicity. Remember, your planned maximum depth may be shallower than the depth at which you reach 1.4 based on other limits, such as previous dives, environmental conditions, your and your buddy's training and experience, etc.

Maximum and Contingency Depth Table

Blend	Maximum Depth (1.4)	Contingency Depth (1.6)
29%	38 m/126 ft	45 m/149 ft
30%	37 m/121 ft	43 m/143 ft
31%	35 m/116 ft	42 m/137 ft
32%	34 m/111 ft	40 m/132 ft
33%	32 m/107 ft	38 m/127 ft
34%	31 m/103 ft	37 m/122 ft
35%	30 m/99 ft	36 m/118 ft
36%	29 m/95 ft	34 m/114 ft
37%	28 m/92 ft	33 m/110 ft
38%	27 m/89 ft	32 m/106 ft
39%	26 m/85 ft	31m/102 ft
40%	25 m/83 ft	30 m/99 ft

Note: Blends with 28% oxygen or less are not shown because they have maximum depths deeper than the 40 metre/130 foot depth limit for recreational diving.

Your EANx dive computer tracks your oxygen exposure, including surface interval credit, throughout the diving day much as it tracks your exposure to nitrogen. (See manufacturer literature for specifics on how it determines and displays limits and remaining dive times.) When making repetitive dives, when you enter the scroll

mode, your computer will display the shorter of your no decompression limit or oxygen exposure time remaining. Most computers also display your oxygen exposure status as a graph or other indicator in the surface (between dives) mode. In recreational no stop diving, oxygen exposure rarely limits your dive time unless you spend a lot of time near the 1.4 bar/ata PO_2 limit for the blend you're using. Nonetheless, pay attention to your oxygen exposure because it can limit your dive.

Since you want to stay well within oxygen limits, it's recommended that you have a surface interval of at least one hour between enriched air dives whenever possible, especially if you exceed more than 50 percent of your computer's allowable exposure. This is believed to further reduce the likelihood of oxygen toxicity. If your planned dives would cause you to approach or exceed oxygen exposure limits, switch to an enriched air with less oxygen and/or plan your dives to shallower depths.

If you accidentally exceed the maximum oxygen exposure limits for your computer, ascend immediately but slowly, make a safety stop and end the dive. Do not dive for 24 hours, or as stipulated by the computer manufacturer.

Logging Oxygen Exposure

Because different computers display oxygen exposure differently, logging oxygen exposure after a dive depends upon your dive computer. Some display percent of oxygen exposure used, while others give you a more general indication such as bars on a graph. Therefore, you may have a precise number to log, or a more general approximation. It depends upon how the computer provides the information.

Exercise 3

1. Oxygen partial pressure (check all that apply):

   ☐ a. is used to measure the concentration of oxygen a diver is exposed to.

   ☐ b. expresses the part of a gas pressure exerted by the oxygen in the gas.

   ☐ c. is usually expressed in "atmospheres," abbreviated "ata" or in bar.

   ☐ d. will vary at a given depth depending upon the oxygen percent.

2. Exposure to increased oxygen partial pressure can make your allowable dive time:

   ☐ a. unchanged.

   ☐ b. longer.

   ☐ c. shorter.

   ☐ d. There's not enough information to answer the question.

3. The maximum and contingency oxygen partial pressure limits are:

   ☐ a. 1.4 ata/bar and 1.7 ata/bar

   ☐ b. 1.1 ata/bar and 1.6 ata/bar

   ☐ c. 1.1 ata/bar and 1.4 ata/bar

   ☐ d. 1.4 ata/bar and 1.6 ata/bar

4. The primary hazard of exceeding the oxygen exposure limits is:

   ☐ a. nausea.

   ☐ b. decompression illness.

   ☐ c. a fatal accident due to convulsing and drowning.

   ☐ d. facial twitching.

5. Signs and symptoms that may precede a convulsion due to oxygen toxicity include (check all that apply):

   ☐ a. visual disturbances.

   ☐ b. ear ringing.

   ☐ c. dizziness.

   ☐ d. limb and joint pain.

6. If you experience symptoms of oxygen toxicity, you should ascend immediately and end the dive.

   ☐ True   ☐ False

7. You use your EANx dive computer to manage oxygen exposure by (check all that apply):

   ☐ a. setting its maximum PO_2 at 1.4.

   ☐ b. staying well within its oxygen limits and above the maximum depth for the blend you're using.

   ☐ c. avoiding heavy exercise and carbon dioxide buildup.

   ☐ d. maintaining good buoyancy and depth control.

8. If you accidentally exceed the oxygen exposure limits for your computer, you should (check all that apply):

   ☐ a. ascend immediately but slowly and end the dive.

   ☐ b. skip the safety stop.

   ☐ c. not dive for 24 hours, or as stipulated by the manufacturer.

   ☐ d. clear your computer's memory.

How did you do?

1. *a, b, c, d.* 2. *c. Diving with enriched air usually gives you longer dive times due to reduced nitrogen, but at times oxygen exposure can limit your dive time.* 3. *d.* 4. *c.* 5. *a, b, c.* 6. *True.* 7. *a, b, c, d.* 8. *a, c.*

Oxygen Analysis and Obtaining *Enriched Air Fills*

Checking and Confirming What Blend You're Diving

Study Objectives

Underline/highlight the answers to these questions as you read:

1. Who must personally verify the analysis of the oxygen content in an enriched air cylinder before it is used?

2. What are the procedures for analyzing enriched air?

3. What is standard of practice for the accuracy of enriched air analysis?

4. What cylinder marking should you check to compare your analysis against?

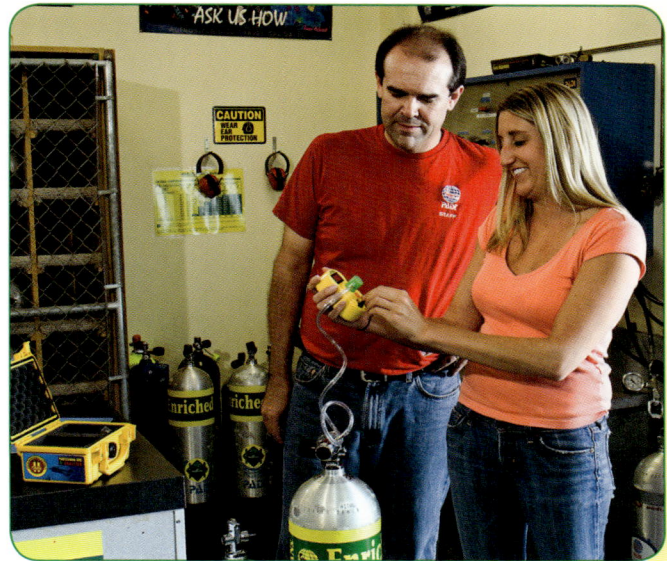

Enriched air fills and rental protocols are important in managing some of the potential problems when diving with enriched air nitrox. These protocols begin when you visit an enriched air fill station, where you'll be asked to show your PADI Enriched Air Diver certification.

After showing your certification, you'll ask for the blend of enriched air you want, although in some cases they'll tell you what they have available. If you want anything else, you may have to wait while they blend. Dive boats – especially live-aboards – that offer enriched air fills onboard may only have a single blend available; if so, it's usually one well-suited to the dive sites they visit. Some dive operations will bring filled enriched air cylinders to the dive site for their sponsored dive trips and travel – either they'll bring the appropriate blend (such as if you're in training), or you let them know what you'd like ahead of time.

Oxygen Analysis

Regardless of how it's blended or where you obtain it, before diving with a cylinder of enriched air nitrox you must analyze it to confirm the percentage of oxygen. You need to know the percentage so you can set your enriched air dive computer, and you must be sure that the oxygen percentage is what the blender says it is.

When making enriched air, the blender analyzes the enriched air to determine the oxygen content. The blender records the information in the fill log and on a sticker (decal) or tag on the cylinder. **Even though the blender analyzes the fill, you must personally verify the oxygen analysis of the cylinder. Do not dive with a cylinder of enriched air if you have not personally verified its contents. There are no exceptions.**

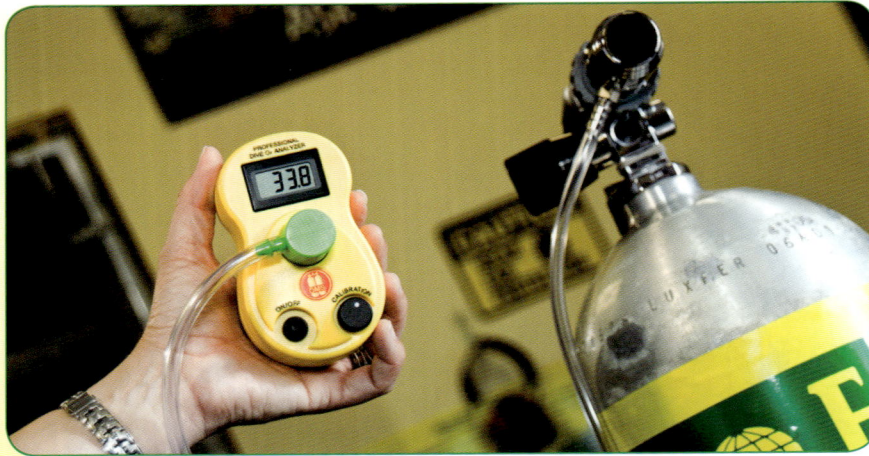

Do not dive with a cylinder of enriched air if you have not personally verified its contents. There are no exceptions.

Usually you'll simply analyze the cylinder contents yourself, but sometimes another qualified person performs the analysis while you watch and *personally* verify the oxygen content on the oxygen analyzer. Ideally, analyze with a different analyzer from the one the blender used – but this isn't always practical nor is it critical.

Decompression sickness (DCS) or drowning due to oxygen toxicity become very real risks if a cylinder contains an enriched air blend different from what you believe it to be. Personally checking is an important safety principle; it double checks the initial analysis, verifies that the cylinder has been correctly marked for that blend and confirms the cylinder wasn't accidentally confused with another.

No matter how competent and well-intentioned someone may be, don't accept the analysis of another individual. It's *your* safety at stake. The consequences of an error will affect you. This is why the dive community standard is that it's *your responsibility* to know what blend you're diving by *personally* confirming it.

Again, some perspective is important. Errors are rare, and you may make hundreds of enriched air dives without ever finding a significant difference between

your analysis and the blender's. *But, it has happened.* Cylinders have been confused and mismarked, and it was the diver's personal analysis that caught the error.

It's important to avoid the possibility of someone else using and refilling the cylinder without your knowledge between when you analyze it and when you dive it. It's also important that the cylinder hasn't accidentally become confused with another.

This isn't usually difficult. This is one reason why your name is on an enriched air cylinder you will use. Keep the cylinder where it won't be used accidentally by someone else. And, **if there's ever any question about an enriched air cylinder's contents, or whether cylinders may have been confused, reanalyze the contents before diving with it.**

If a buddy obtained your cylinder or had it filled for you or the dive operation delivers the cylinder to the dive site, you'll need to personally verify the cylinder contents at the dive site. Again, if you've not personally analyzed it, you don't dive it. It's also a good practice to reanalyze your cylinder contents just before the dive, such as when hooking up your gear.

Using an Oxygen Analyzer

Whether you perform the oxygen analysis yourself or watch a qualified person do it, you need to know how to analyze properly.

Oxygen analyzers come in different sizes and types; some read out digitally and others use analog (needle) gauges. Whatever type, for analyzing enriched air you need one that reads to one-tenth of a percent. Different

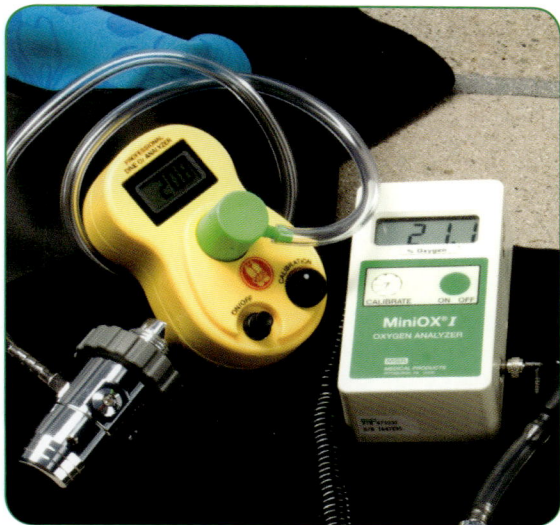

Oxygen analyzers come in different sizes and types; some read out digitally and others use analog (needle) gauges. Whatever type, for analyzing enriched air you need one that reads to one-tenth of a percent.

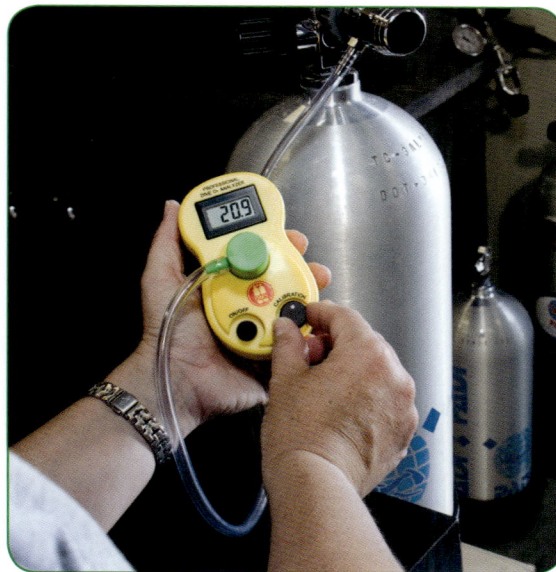

The preferred method for calibrating an analyzer is to use a flow meter or flow restrictor to flow air (not enriched air) from a scuba cylinder slowly across the analyzer's sensor. Turn the calibration knob until the analyzer reads 20.8% to 21% as specified by the manufacturer.

types and models of analyzers have their unique features, but in general, the following steps apply (your instructor will have you practice these steps, and be sure to consult the manufacturer literature for the particular model or models you use):

1. *Turn the analyzer on.* An oxygen analyzer usually needs to be calibrated each time it's turned on. The simplest method is to calibrate for air.

   The preferred method is to have air (not enriched air) from a scuba cylinder flow slowly across the analyzer's sensor at a controlled rate. There are inexpensive flow meters and flow restrictors you can use. Some analyzers have built-in flow devices that let you simply hold the end against the cylinder valve (just barely flowing) for calibration (and analysis). Use about the same flow rate that you'll analyze with. Turn the calibration knob until the analyzer reads 20.8% to 21% as specified by the manufacturer.

2. *Flow the enriched air you're analyzing into the analyzer at the same rate you used for calibration.* (A higher or lower rate may create inaccuracy.) Give enough time to clear any air in the valve, lines and flow device. (Note: When opening the valve on an enriched air cylinder, open the valve *slowly*. This reduces the heat associated with rapid pressurization, helping minimize oxygen fire concerns.) Read the oxygen percentage from the analyzer display.

   EANx that was mixed using partial pressure blending in your cylinder may need some time to mix evenly to get an accurate reading. Rolling the cylinder back and forth speeds this up, but most divers simply let it sit for 30 minutes to an hour before analyzing. Banked, continuous flow or membrane blended enriched air will be ready to analyze immediately.

3. *Don't blow into the sensor because your breath contains moisture, which affects accuracy and reduces the sensor life.* Store your analyzer in a cool place with low humidity.

4. *Check your analyzer periodically against other analyzers and replace its sensor if it performs outside the tolerance levels specified by the manufacturer, and at intervals specified by the manufacturer.*

5. *If you ever question the accuracy of an analyzer, compare it against one or more analyzers known to be accurate, and/or a gas of known analysis.* Consult the manufacturer's instructions about ensuring accuracy. Don't use the unit until you confirm that it is accurate.

Blend accuracy. The standard of practice for enriched air is plus or minus 1%. Minor variations (less than 1%) between the blender's analysis and yours are normal, but a substantial variation should be confirmed by using another analyzer. Most enriched air computers use 1 percent increments. Round up or down to the closest whole percent (e.g., round 31.2 percent to 31 percent and 31.8 percent to 32 percent), unless the computer manufacturer literature has a different recommendation.

Stickers, Tags, Decals and the Fill Log

After analyzing the cylinder contents, compare your analysis with the contents tag or sticker on the cylinder. In some cases, the sticker or tag may already be partially completed, and you verify and finish filling it out. At a busy blending station, you may fill it out entirely and attach it to your cylinder.

There are different versions of content stickers (decals)/tags, but as you learned earlier, the fill sticker or tag lists, at a minimum, your final analyzed oxygen content, the fill date, the maximum depth to which the blend can be used (i.e.,as previously

Own Your Own Analyzer

Although most enriched air dive operations have oxygen analyzers you can use when you obtain enriched air, most divers certified to use nitrox prefer to own their own. If you're serious about diving with enriched air, you'll find it's definitely worth investing in one.

- You can analyze enriched air any time, not just in a dive operation, which can be especially handy if a contents question comes up at a dive site.

- Since you maintain the analyzer, you can be sure that it's accurate and that the sensor is replaced as required.

- When several divers have analyzers, there are always two or three others with which to compare if there are accuracy questions.

- At a busy enriched air fill center, having your own analyzer saves time because you don't have to wait to use the dive center's.

- After you invest in your own analyzer, remember that you have to replace the sensor periodically. This is a minor expense that you only have to make every one to three years.

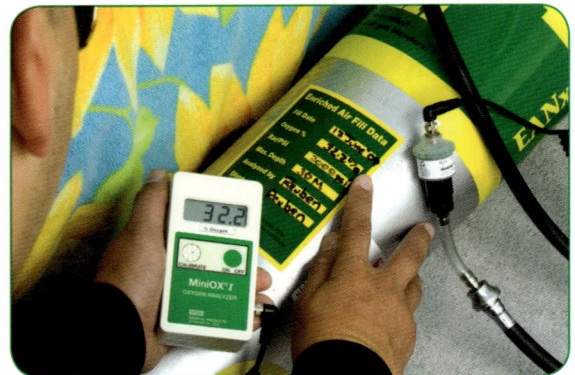

After analyzing the cylinder contents, compare your analysis with the contents tag or sticker on the cylinder. If there is ever any doubt about a cylinder's contents, reanalyze it before diving with it.

1.4) and the diver/final analyzer's name. You may also find a place for the fill pressure and the blender's initial analysis.

After you've used the cylinder, *leave the sticker in place*. The blender will remove it when refilling the cylinder. The sticker tells the blender the oxygen content of the remaining enriched air.

Some divers and dive operations prefer tags or reusable stickers. If tags are used, be sure that the cylinder serial number on the tag matches the actual serial number on the cylinder. After using an enriched air cylinder, some divers write "empty" on the sticker or tag so that the cylinder isn't mistaken for one that is full.

When having an empty enriched air cylinder filled, don't worry about the remaining enriched air in the cylinder. The blender will release it if necessary; don't drain it because it may not be necessary. And, the blender may analyze the contents to confirm the cylinder wasn't improperly refilled.

After checking and completing (as necessary) the

contents sticker/tag, you'll also sign the enriched air fill station's fill log. In many cases, the fill log takes the form of a statement of understanding that you sign.

At a minimum, the fill log lists the cylinder serial number, the date, the blender's analysis, the maximum depth for the blend and the diver's name and signature. The log may record other information, depending upon the needs of the operation. If you get the cylinder at the dive site, the dive operation will bring a fill log to complete and sign on location.

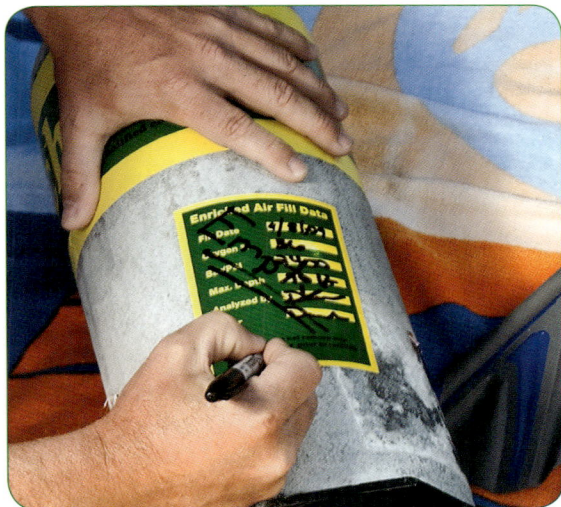

After you've used the cylinder, leave the sticker in place. Some divers write "empty" on the sticker or tag so that the cylinder isn't mistaken for one that is full.

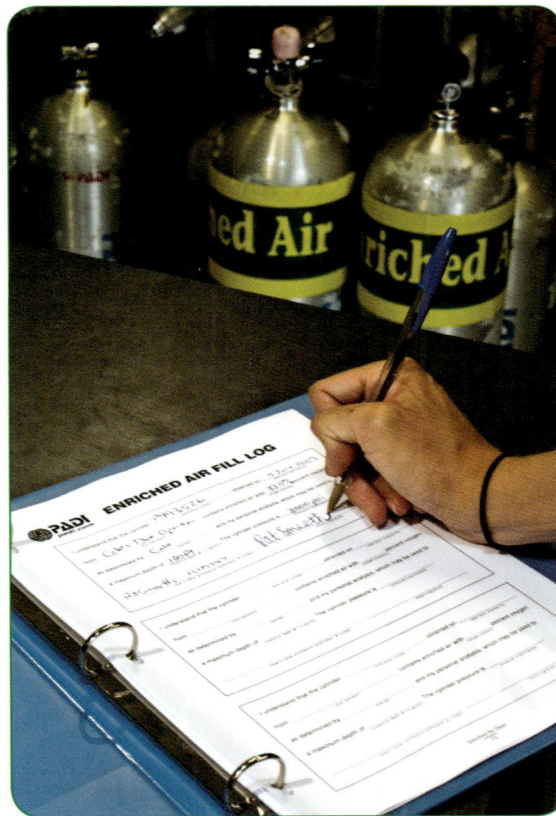

After checking and completing (as necessary) the contents sticker/tag, you'll also sign the enriched air fill station's fill log. At a minimum, the fill log lists the tank serial number, the date, the blender's analysis, the maximum depth for the blend and the diver's name and signature.

Exercise 4

1. Who must personally verify the analysis of the oxygen content in an enriched air cylinder before it is used?

   ☐ a. The divemaster in charge
   ☐ b. The boat captain
   ☐ c. The diver who will use the cylinder
   ☐ d. The buddy of the diver who will use the cylinder

2. The first step in analyzing enriched air is to calibrate the oxygen analyzer.

   ☐ True   ☐ False

3. The standard of practice for the accuracy of enriched air analysis is plus or minus

   ☐ a. 0%   ☐ c. 2%
   ☐ b. 1%   ☐ d. 3%

4. After analyzing enriched air, you should compare the oxygen percent with

   ☐ a. the blender's guidelines.
   ☐ b. the percentage marked on the contents sticker or tag.
   ☐ c. the calibration percent.
   ☐ d. None of the above.

How did you do?

1. *c.* **2.** *True.* **3.** *b.* **4.** *b.*

Guidelines for Diving with Enriched Air
Dive Computers
Using Technology for Maximum Effect

Study Objectives

Underline/highlight the answers to these questions as you read:

1. What four guidelines apply to diving with an enriched air dive computer?

2. How do you set your enriched air dive computer?

3. What happens if you forget to set your enriched air computer before a dive?

4. What should you do if your enriched air dive computer fails during a dive?

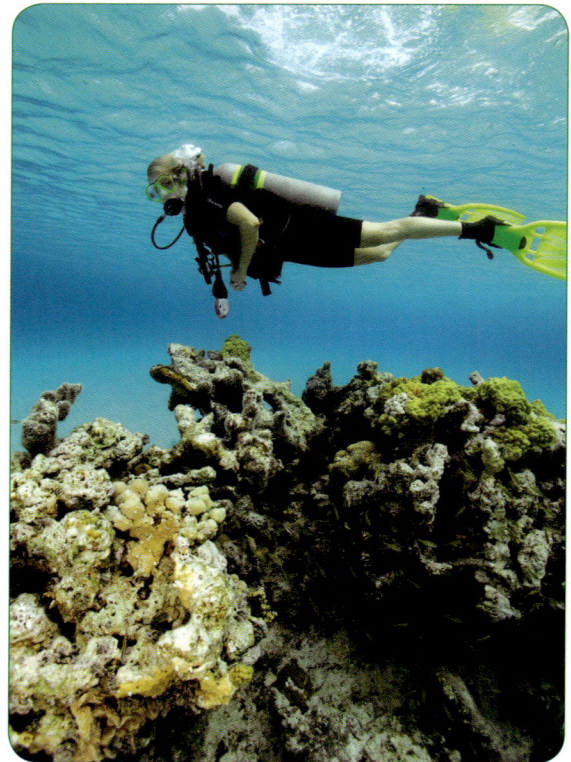

Four Guidelines

Today, most serious divers use dive computers – whether they're diving air or enriched air. There are four guidelines to apply when diving with an enriched air dive computer:

1. Know the EANx blend's maximum depth and stay shallower by watching the depth display. Remember to plan your dive, and dive your plan. Use the maximum depth warning as a *secondary* alert.

2. As you already learned as an Open Water Diver, stay well within your computer's limits. With EANx, this means staying well within both the no stop and oxygen exposure limits. Watch both displays on your computer. If you begin to near a limit, ascend until your computer displays a longer limit. Stay that shallow or shallower for the rest of the dive.

3. Each diver should have an individual enriched air dive computer set for the blend the diver is using. Variations in depths as well as any variations in the blends will result in differences in the no stop times and oxygen exposure the computers calculate. As you would when diving air, stay within the limits of whichever buddy's computer gives the most conservative readings.

4. Make safety stops and follow all the conservative diving practices you've already learned.

Each diver should have an individual enriched air computer set for the blend the diver's using. And, you should make safety stops and follow all the conservative diving practices you've already learned when using nitrox.

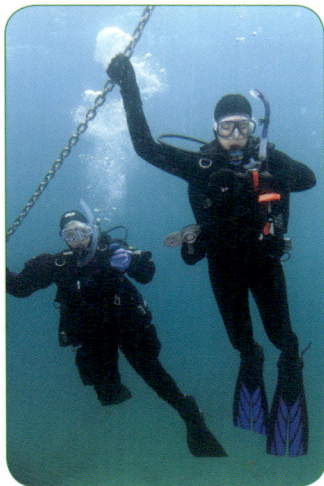

Setting an Enriched Air Dive Computer

Earlier, you learned that before each dive, you set your dive computer for the oxygen percent of the enriched air blend you'll be using. This allows the computer to calculate your no stop time and your oxygen exposure. Let's look at this in more detail.

How you set the oxygen percent varies from model to model. Generally, you enter a "set" mode by pressing a button or touching electrical contacts. Typically, you can tell you're in the set mode when the oxygen percentage number blinks, indicating it's waiting for you to change it.

Next, you scroll the percentage, usually in 1% increments, to the blend you're using (remember to round to the closest 1% from your analysis) and lock it in. Most computers scroll the percentage by either holding a button or maintaining a contact continuously. When you reach the desired percentage, you release the button or contacts, then lock the setting by pressing a button or another set of contacts. With most computers, the oxygen percent stops flashing when you've locked it in. Your instructor and/or the manufacturer instructions will explain how to do this with your specific model, and you'll do this before each dive during the course.

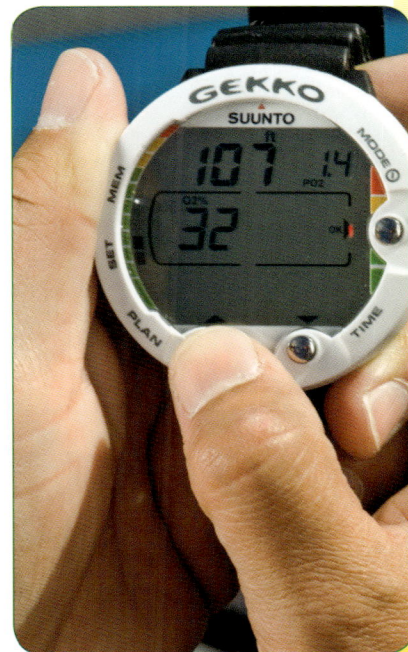

How you set the oxygen percent varies from model to model. Generally, you enter a "set" mode by pressing a button or electrical contacts. Typically, you can tell you're in the set mode when the oxygen percentage number blinks, indicating it's waiting for you to change it.

After you've done it a couple of times, it will be second nature.

After an enriched air dive, some computers will clear their settings and wait for you to reset them before you dive again. If you forget, these go into some kind of error mode. One common error mode is to default to a worst-case impossible mix of 79% nitrogen, 50% oxygen, which causes the computer to severely limit your no stop time. Other computers remain set for the last blend you used until you change it. The thinking is that it's common to dive the same blend for multiple dives and divers know it's important to reset their computers if they change blend. Keeping the blend set avoids unnecessary resetting when diving the same EANx for multiple dives. Some of these types will go into an error or warning mode if you don't dive for 12 to 24 hours and then forget to set the blend, but not all models. Be sure to consult the manufacturer literature so you know if and when your computer clears the blend settings after a dive. In any event, remember that failing to have your computer set for the EANx blend raises the risk of DCS or oxygen toxicity.

An exception is if you set it for air (21%). When set for air, virtually all computers stay set for air, dive after dive, until you change it.

If Your Computer Fails

Dive computers are very reliable, and failures are very rare. Nonetheless, if your computer fails during a dive, immediately ascend, make a safety stop at 5 metres/15 feet for 3 minutes or longer and end the dive.

An option that's growing in popularity is to wear a backup (second) EANx computer. This lets you continue the dive and make repetitive dives if your primary computer fails. Many divers who do this invest in a less expensive secondary computer that calculates similarly to their primary (usually the same brand), two identical computers, or a computer-watch (a dive computer that is also and the size of a digital watch). The primary (and very minor) downside is having to set two computers prior to each dive.

Another option is to keep a written record of EANx blends (e.g. in your log book), maximum depths, bottom times and surface intervals throughout the day. If your computer fails (during or between dives), you can use tables to calculate your no stop limits and oxygen exposure and continue diving. (See your instructor to learn more about using enriched air and oxygen exposure tables.)

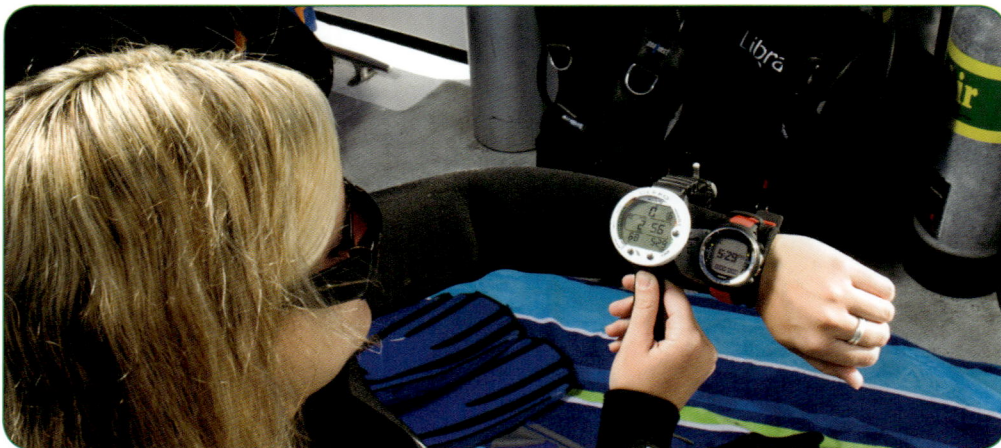

Dive computers are very reliable and failures are rare. Nonetheless, many divers wear a backup so they can continue diving in the event their primary computer fails.

If you weren't wearing a backup computer and tables aren't an option, do not dive for at least 12 hours (or longer if specified by the manufacturer) before resuming with a working dive computer.

Using an Air-Only Computer

It's possible to dive with EANx using an air-only (not enriched air compatible) computer. You may want to do this because you only have such a computer and only EANx (not air) available. Also, when using enriched air within air no stop limits, you can get closer to the limits without "pushing" them. You may therefore opt for enriched air for a dive that may approach your air computer's no decompression limits. However, even when using EANx, you should stay *well within* the computer's limits and avoid diving *to* them.

Besides losing the extended no stop time you would have with an EANx compatible computer, a drawback to using an air-only computer is that it doesn't track your oxygen exposure. You can accommodate this one of two ways. The first way is more versatile with respect to your choice of blends, depths and allowable time. The second way is more limiting, but much simpler and adequate for many diving circumstances.

Option 1. Use the DSAT Equivalent Air Depth and Oxygen Exposure Tables.

Using these tables, you determine your maximum depth (PO_2 of 1.4 bar/ata), as well as track your oxygen exposure based on the deepest depth you actually reach during each dive. If you're interested in learning to do this, your instructor can show you how to use these tables.

Option 2. Stay within these limits:

- Use an EANx blend with 32% or less oxygen.

- Limit your depth to 30 metres/100 feet.

- Stay within your computer's no decompression limits.

- Limit your total dive time for the entire day to 160 minutes.

Staying within these limits will keep you above the maximum depth for the blend and within accepted oxygen exposure limits.

Exercise 5

1. When diving with an enriched air computer (check all that apply):

   ☐ a. It's acceptable for a buddy team to share a single computer.

   ☐ b. Stay well within the computer's no stop and oxygen exposure limits.

   ☐ c. Make safety stops and follow all the conservative diving practices you've already learned.

   ☐ d. Know the blend's maximum depth and rely on the computer warning as a secondary alert only.

2. You set most enriched air computers by letting the computer automatically analyze the blend you're using.

   ☐ True   ☐ False

3. If you forget to set your enriched air computer before a dive (check all that apply)

   ☐ a. the computer enters an error mode.

   ☐ b. the computer will select the most common blend used in the area.

   ☐ c. you may have to wait 12 hours before you use it again.

4. If your enriched air dive computer fails during a dive

   ☐ a. share your buddy's computer for the rest of the dive.

   ☐ b. ascend immediately, make a safety stop at 5 metres/15 Feet and end the dive.

How did you do?

1. b, c, d. 2. False. Computers do not analyze your gas blend. You have to set the computer based on your analysis. 3. a, c. 4. b.

Diving Emergencies and *Enriched Air*

PADI Rescue Diver Manual, Emergency First Response *Primary and Secondary Care Participant* Manual, PADI *Emergency Oxygen Provider Manual*

Just in Case

Study Objectives

Underline/highlight the answers to these questions as you read:

1. What action should you take if a diver convulses underwater?

2. What action should you take if a diver is suspected of having decompression illness after a dive using enriched air?

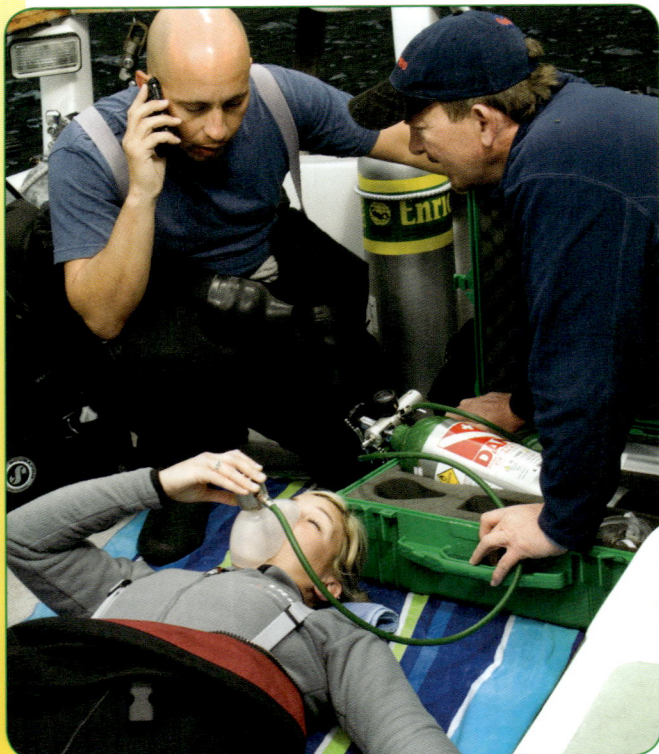

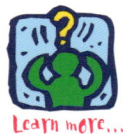

Oxygen Toxicity

Assuming you and your dive partners follow the accepted guidelines for diving with enriched air nitrox, it's very unlikely that you'll have to assist a diver with oxygen toxicity.

However, if a diver convulses underwater due to oxygen toxicity – or any other reason for that matter – the generally recommended action is to handle the emergency as you would for any unresponsive diver underwater: If the diver's mouthpiece is in place, hold it there, but don't waste time trying to replace it if it's not. Immediately surface the diver, establish ample positive buoyancy for yourself and the victim, and check for breathing. Call for assistance if available and begin in-water rescue breaths if the victim isn't breathing. Get the diver to the boat or shore and from the water as quickly as possible without jeopardizing your own safety.

Once out of the water, check for a heart beat and breathing. If they're absent, begin/continue rescue breaths and/or CPR. In any case, activate local Emergency Medical Services (EMS). If the diver is breathing, begin first aid for DCI as a precaution. Even if apparently fully recovered, the diver should be examined by a physician.

This recommendation is based on the US Navy procedures, which the Divers Alert Network defers to. There hasn't been much study of this because such a study would be dangerous to the subjects, nor have there been many incidents upon which to base a formal protocol.

Some experts recommend that if the diver's mouthpiece is in, hold it in place and wait to begin the ascent until after the convulsion subsides. Then surface the diver immediately. This recommendation is based on the concern that a convulsing diver may not breathe regularly. Regardless, the primary concern is getting the diver to the surface to prevent drowning, and so you can begin first aid and get help. Recommendations for handling an underwater convulsion may change as information becomes available. Stay informed and follow the current recommendations.

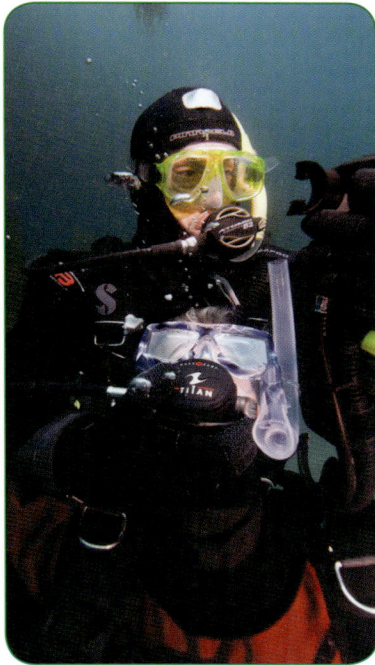

If a diver convulses underwater due to oxygen toxicity – or any other reason for that matter – the generally recommended action is to handle the emergency as you would for any unresponsive diver underwater: If the diver has the mouthpiece in place, hold it there; but don't waste time trying to replace it if it's not. Immediately bring the diver to the surface and check for breathing.

Decompression Illness

Divers commonly ask if there's any difference in the way you would handle a suspected DCI emergency for a diver who had been using enriched air versus for one who had been using air. The answer is "no." If a diver is suspected of having DCI after an enriched air or an air dive, administer oxygen, and provide first aid as necessary. Get the diver into the care of the appropriate local EMS, and contact the Divers Alert Network office that serves your area.

When possible, tell emergency personnel the particulars about the diver's dive profile, including depth, time and whether the diver was using a dive computer or tables. This information would also include whether the diver was using air or, if using enriched air, what the blend was. In a DCI emergency, if you run out of emergency oxygen before you can get a responsive patient into emergency medical care, have the patient breathe any enriched air available. While not as beneficial as 100% oxygen, enriched air has more oxygen than air and may help. It certainly won't hurt. For an unresponsive patient, at least one manufacturer makes a system that allows you to provide EANx from a scuba cylinder, much as you provide oxygen from an emergency oxygen system.

You can learn more about handling emergencies by completing the Emergency First Response, Primary Care (CPR) and Secondary Care (First Aid) courses and the PADI Rescue Diver and Emergency Oxygen Provider courses.

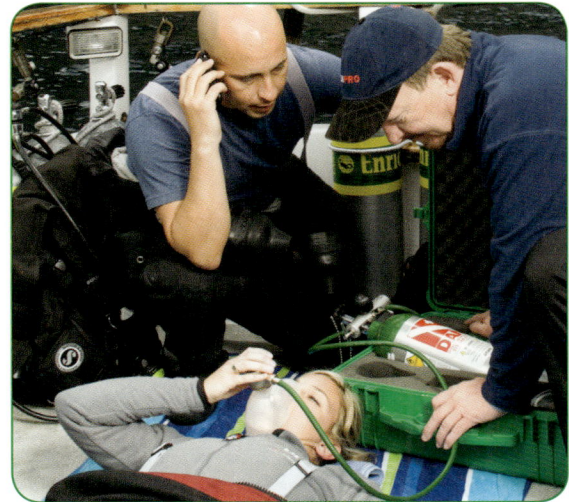

If a diver is suspected of having DCI after an enriched air or air dive, administer oxygen, and provide first aid as necessary. Get the diver into the care of the appropriate local EMS, and contact the Divers Alert Network office that serves your area.

What's in the Cylinder You Hang?

If you've completed the PADI Advanced Open Water Diver course, you already know that when making dives deeper than 18 metres/60 feet, if circumstances make it reasonably feasible, it's a good idea to hang a contingency cylinder and regulator with extra air or enriched air at 5 metres/15 feet. This ensures that you have enough air for a safety stop or emergency decompression stop.

This sometimes raises a question: If you're diving with enriched air, what should be in that cylinder? Air? Enriched air? How about a different blend from the one you're using?

It depends.

Your computer's calculations assume you're breathing the enriched air blend you programmed into it. If

you switch to air or an enriched air blend with less oxygen than you used during the dive, you'll be releasing nitrogen more slowly than the computer believes. This may affect the accuracy of repetitive dives, and in the case of emergency decompression, could mean your emergency stop is too short.

If you switch to a blend with *more* oxygen than the one you used during the dive, you don't negatively affect your repetitive dive no stop time calculations or emergency decompression calculations. Technically, it affects the oxygen exposure calculations, but since oxygen exposure is minimal during a three to five minute stop at 5 metres/15 feet (with up to EANx40), this shouldn't be a problem as long

as you remain well within your computer's oxygen limits.

So, one option is to be sure the hang cylinder has the same or more oxygen than what you make the dive with. But, many enriched air computers offer you a second option: programming for two or more blends. Although intended primarily for tec diving, if your computer allows you to switch gases during the dive, you can have it set for both your dive blend *and* the hang cylinder blend so you can switch in a contingency situation.

Computers vary in how they perform their calculations, so it's best to consult the manufacturer's instructions for particulars about safety stops and emergency decompression stops.

Exercise 6

1. If a diver using enriched air convulses underwater, you should attempt to give the diver regular air from a pony bottle.

☐ True   ☐ False

2. If a diver is suspected of having DCI after a dive using enriched air, you should (check all that apply):

☐ a. Handle the situation as you normally would, except don't give emergency oxygen.
☐ b. Recompress the diver in the water.
☐ c. Contact local emergency personnel and diver emergency services.
☐ d. Administer emergency oxygen and first aid as you normally would.

How did you do?

1. *False. You should treat the situation as an unresponsive diver underwater emergency and bring the diver to the surface.* **2.** *c, d.*

Practical Applications and
Enriched Air Training Dives

As part of the PADI Enriched Air Diver course, you will complete two Practical Applications. Your instructor may schedule them together into a single class meeting.

During Practical Application I, you'll learn to use one or more oxygen analyzers. Besides learning how to confirm what EANx blend a cylinder has, you'll determine the maximum depth and check that the cylinder markings correctly reflect the blend and the depth.

During Practical Application II, you'll go through all the steps that a typical enriched air fill station has in practice when obtaining enriched air. You'll request a specific EANx blend, analyze it, confirm cylinder markings and sign the station's fill log. Your instructor may also give you a tour and provide an overview of how they blend enriched air.

During the Enriched Air Training Dives, under instructor supervision, you'll practice predive cylinder analysis, setting your EANx compatible dive computer, establishing maximum depths and all the other steps involved with planning enriched air dives.

In some situations, your instructor may have you complete two predive simulations instead of actual training dives. This isn't as much fun as actually diving, but you learn what you need to know because the key steps to EANx diving are in the predive planning. Once you have your gas analyzed and your computer set, the dive is easy — you simply stay within the limits you set when you planned the dive, and well within computer limits.

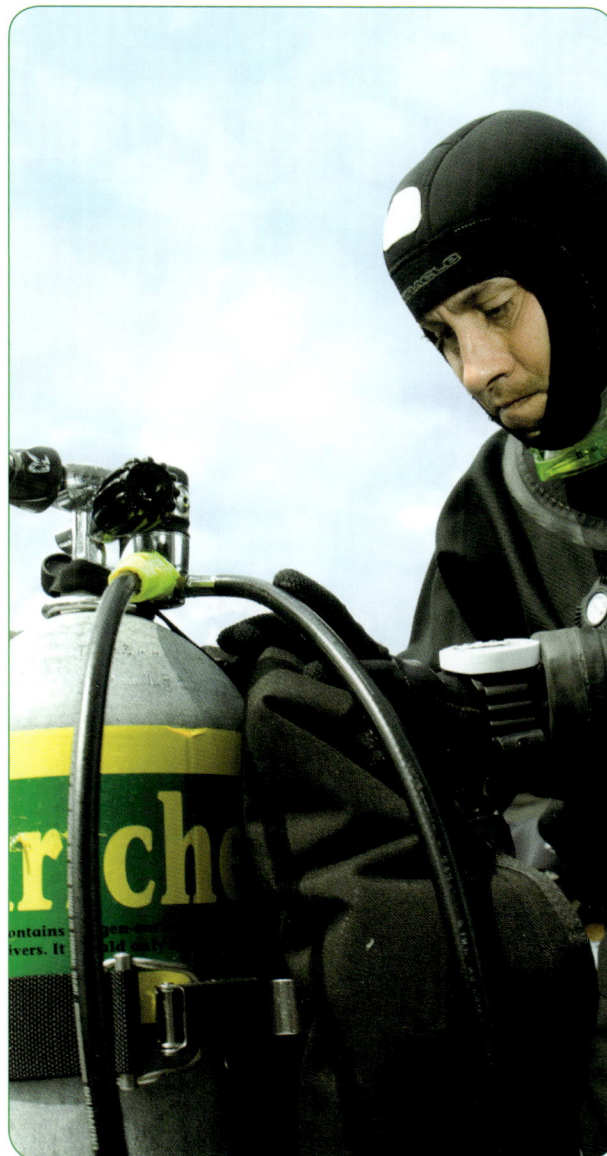

Knowledge Review –
Enriched Air Diver

1. What is the primary benefit of using enriched air nitrox? What advantages does this provide?

LESS NITROGEN EXPOSURE. PROLONGED DIVE TIME.

2. How does using EANx affect narcosis while diving?

NO DIFFERENT TO AN AIR DIVE.

3. What is the primary concern regarding enriched air nitrox and equipment? What are recommendations for using equipment, other than cylinders, with enriched air with up to 40% oxygen? (Consider local regulations in your response, if appropriate.)

NO MODIFICATIONS.

4. What is the potential hazard of improper enriched air filling procedures?

enriched air should not be put in a regular air cylinder because of the risk of explosion.

5. List the markings that, according to broadly accepted dive community practices, you should have on a scuba cylinder used for enriched air nitrox. Are these markings used everywhere?

10cm banded reading "NITROX" (yellow cylinder)
15 cm banned — " — (non-yellow clynder).

6. What are the oxygen partial pressures of the maximum and contingency depth limits for a given enriched air blend? What is the primary hazard of exceeding oxygen limits? How do you avoid the hazard?

1.4 bar
cont. 1.6 bar.

7. What signs and symptoms may precede a CNS convulsion? Do these always precede a convulsion?

tunnel vison, ears ringing, nausea, twitching

VENTED.

8. Describe how to use an EANx compatible dive computer to remain within accepted oxygen exposure limits. What should you do if you accidentally exceed the oxygen limits of your computer?

Set 1.4 as max, Set oxy blend. record max depth for 1.4 bar of oxy blend. if exceed 1.4 bar end dive and ascend slowly.

9. Who must personally verify the oxygen analysis of a cylinder of enriched air? What is the procedure for doing this?

check your own cylinder. oxygen meter on air tank calibrate 20.8% to 21% then compare to enriched air.

10. What should you do if your enriched air computer fails during a dive?

immediately ascend with a safety stop at 5m. note. air%/max depth and bottom times.

11. What should you do if a diver convulses underwater?

ascending, positive buoyancy, rescue breaths, to boat or shore, first aid / call 999.

12. What should you do for a diver suspected of having decompression illness after an enriched air dive?

call ems.

Student Statement: I've reviewed the questions and answers, and for any I answered incorrectly or incompletely, I now understand what I missed.

Name _Avert_ Date _01/04/2013._

35

Appendix
Enriched Air at Altitude

If you're familiar with diving at altitude procedures, you're probably aware that your theoretical depth at altitudes above 300 metres/1000 feet is deeper than your actual depth. You use this theoretical depth for dive planning with the RDP in place of your real depth. In addition, many dive computers can be set (or set themselves) to adjust for altitude. Either way, altitude reduces your allowable no stop time for a given depth.

This causes some divers to ask, "Can I use enriched air nitrox at altitude to cancel out the effect of the theoretical depth?"

That's a really good question, but at this writing there aren't any really good answers. Basically, it boils down to these two facts:

- It works in theory, and there's nothing in the calculations that says it shouldn't work, but . . .

- . . . despite theory, there's not been much formal testing of the concept.

It's well known that quite a few divers do use enriched air nitrox to offset the reduced no stop times you have at altitude. Some (perhaps most) enriched air dive computers will calculate EANx dives at altitude (see the manufacturer literature for your particular model). Nonetheless, the hyperbaric medical community has not formally recognized the practice as acceptable –

not because of a known problem, but because there's neither extensive research nor a quantifiable experience data base to support the practice.

Until such data emerge, the only recommendation the dive community can make is that you can use enriched air at altitude as though you were diving air with respect to no stop limits, but calculate oxygen exposure for the enriched air blend you're using. This means setting your dive computer as though diving air, and calculating your oxygen exposure using tables such as the DSAT Oxygen Exposure Table (see your PADI Instructor for information about using the DSAT Oxygen Exposure Table). Alternatively, you can dive with one computer set for your enriched air blend and another set for air (and both set for altitude). Stay within the oxygen limits on the one set for nitrox, and within the no decompression limits of the one set for air.

Although using enriched air at altitude may not offer a formally endorsed way to offset the reduced no stop time (at least for now), it does have another benefit: Divers unacclimated to altitude may feel weakened or air-starved at the surface due to the thin air, especially when swimming at the surface or climbing out of the water after the dive. Breathing from a cylinder of enriched air often provides relief, thanks to the higher oxygen content.

DAN *Nitrox Workshop*

The most recent industry-wide workshop took place in November 2000. The major entities involved with recreational enriched air diving met to discuss the issues surrounding enriched air nitrox use and training. The Divers Alert Network sponsored the two-day meeting in Durham, North Carolina, USA, which was chaired by Michael A. Lang of the USA's Smithsonian Institution.

The workshop included papers, presentations and discussion by leaders in dive training, medicine, operations and equipment with respect to enriched air nitrox. Attendees included representatives from PADI and PADI's corporate affiliate, DSAT (Diving Science and Technology).

At the end of the two days, the workshop achieved a dive community consensus with respect to issues regarding the training of recreational enriched air divers, the use of enriched air with modern scuba equipment and some medical questions.

The PADI Enriched Air Diver course follows the community standard consensus this important workshop achieved; consensus findings follow.

For copies of the papers presented and the discussions, contact the Divers Alert Network, 6 West Colony Place, Durham, NC 27710, USA, or your local DAN office for a copy of *DAN Nitrox Workshop Proceedings*, Michael A. Lang, editor.

Consensus Recommendations

For entry-level, recreational open circuit nitrox diving:

- No evidence was presented that showed an increased risk of DCS from the use of oxygen enriched air (nitrox) versus compressed air.

- A maximum PO_2 of 1.6 ata was accepted based on its history of use and scientific studies.

- Routine CO_2 retention screening is not necessary.

- Oxygen analyzers should use a controlled-flow sampling device.

- Oxygen analysis of the breathing gas should be performed by the blender and/or dispenser and verified by the end user.

- Training agencies recognize the effectiveness of dive computers.

- For recreational diving, there is no need to track whole body exposure to oxygen (OTU/UPTD).

- Use of the "CNS Oxygen Clock" concept, based on NOAA oxygen exposure limits, should be taught. However, it should be noted that CNS oxygen toxicity could occur suddenly and unexpectedly. (Note: Virtually all modern EANx computers calculate oxygen exposure based on oxygen "clock," NOAA limits and/or OTU/UPTD.)

- No evidence was presented, based on history of use, to show an unreasonable risk of fire of ignition when using up to 40% nitrox with standard scuba equipment. The level of risk is related to specific equipment configurations and the user should rely on the manufacturer's recommendations.

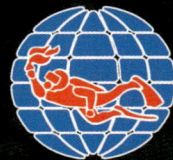

PADI courses have the unique distinction of meeting academic excellence criteria as established by university and vocational accreditation bodies. Find out how you can get credit for your PADI education!

Australia

PADI Divers may receive credit toward various certificates and diplomas for several PADI courses within the Australian national training system. The following training providers recognise certain PADI and Emergency First Response (EFR) courses — Technical and Further Education, South Australia; Australia Fisheries Academy, South Australia; Victorian Tertiary Admissions Center, Victoria; and the Western Australia Curriculum Council. For more information, go to: www.padi.com/scuba/scuba-diving-guide/start-scuba-diving/scuba-lessons-for-college-credit/default.aspx

Canada

The British Columbia Ministry of Education (External Credentials Program for Industrial and Occupational Courses) has approved the PADI Open Water Diver (2 credits), PADI Advanced Open Water or Adventures in Diving Program (4 credits) and PADI Rescue Diver (4 credits) courses for school credit. Grade 10, 11 and 12 students who have been certified in these PADI courses simply present their PADI certification card to the school administration to apply for credit. For information on receiving credit contact your school's administration. On an individual, merit-base case, divers in Canada may also receive credit for PADI courses through the USA-based American Council on Education's College Credit Recommendation Service as noted under "United States."

England, Wales and Northern Ireland

PADI Open Water Scuba Instructors can apply to PADI for the Certificate in Scuba Instruction, a Vocationally Related Qualification (VRQ) accredited at Level 3 on the National Qualifications Framework in England, Wales and Northern Ireland, by the Qualifications and Curriculum Authority (QCA) for England, Department for Education, Lifelong Learning and Skills (DELLS) for Wales and the Council for the Curriculum, Examinations and Assessment (CCEA) for Northern Ireland. The certificate may be accepted by Further Education institutions as proof of eligibility for attendance at higher level courses. Contact ie@padi.co.uk for an application form.

Europe

Divers have received credit for PADI courses in mainland Europe academic institutions and through the military; but since there is no formal recognition process, these have been individual cases. For more information or for a specific request, contact PADI Europe at training@padi.ch

Japan

Those who want to teach diving in Japanese school systems (colleges, universities, vocational schools, etc.) undergo general and specialized course work and testing to become authorized by the Japan Sports Association (JASA), under the jurisdiction of the Ministry of Education, Culture, Sports, Science and Technology. PADI Open Water Scuba Instructors are exempt from this specialized course and test, and can attain JASA authorization by taking a general course and certification test. For more information go to www.japan-sports.or.jp/english

New Zealand

PADI Divers may qualify to receive recognition through a New Zealand Qualification Authority accredited provider. Open Water Diver, Advanced Open Water Diver and Rescue Diver qualify for the National Certificate of Diving: Foundational Skills; Divemasters and Open Water Scuba Instructors qualify for the National Certificate of Diving: Leadership; and Specialty Instructors qualify for the National Certificate of Diving: Instruction. For more information, go to www.padi.com/scuba/scuba-diving-guide/start-scuba-diving/scuba-lessons-for-college-credit/default.aspx

United States

The American Council on Education's College Credit Recommendation Service (ACE CREDIT) has evaluated and recommended college credit for 15 PADI courses, 3 DSAT courses, and 1 Emergency First Response course. The American Council on Education, the major coordinating body for all the nation's higher education institutions, seeks to provide leadership and a unifying voice on key higher education issues and to influence public policy through advocacy, research, and program initiatives. For more information on ACE CREDIT recommendations, and to order an official PADI transcript, go to www.padi.com/scuba/scuba-diving-guide/start-scuba-diving/scuba-lessons-for-college-credit/default.aspx or contact PADI Americas at training@padi.com

NOTES